ACUPUNCTURE ENERGY IN HEALTH AND DISEASE

This textbook for the advanced student of acupuncture provides a clear exposition of the latest theories of energy distribution in the body and gives a detailed summary of treatment, including moxibustion and electronic acupuncture, for a wide range of illnesses and general complaints.

ACUPUNCTURE ENERGY IN HEALTH AND DISEASE

A Practical Guide for Advanced Students

by
**Henry Woollerton and
Colleen J. McLean**

THORSONS PUBLISHERS LIMITED
Wellingborough, Northamptonshire

First published 1979

ISBN 0 7225 0482 9 *(paperback)*
ISBN 0 7225 0521 3 *(hardback)*

Photoset by
Specialised Offset Services Limited, Liverpool
and printed in Great Britain by
Weatherby Woolnough Ltd.,
Sanders Road, Wellingborough, Northamptonshire.

Contents

Introduction

For the student of acupuncture, the first year is the best. It is a time of excitement and discovery. There is no shortage of basic texts which describe 5-element theory, the paths of the Main meridians, the location of the acupuncture points, pulse diagnosis, and *Yin* and *Yang*. These books agree with each other within very close limits.

Unfortunately, this easy start is deceptive. As the student studies further, he is likely to find himself not more enlightened, but more confused. The unanimity amongst the various authorities melts away at about the end of the first text books. The student finds himself on his own trying to make sense, or not, of conflicting translations of Chinese classics, and of widely-opposing opinions as to what is important to the practice of acupuncture.

This book may be thought of as a 'second year' text book. The first part is an attempt to clear a sensible path through a forest of confusion. It deals with the way in which man transforms and utilizes the energy from his environment. It also attempts to clarify and simplify the causes and diagnosis of disease in Chinese terms.

The second part of this book concerns practical treatments. It deals with five forms of treatment:

Needle acupuncture
Electronic stimulation acupuncture
Needleless acupuncture
Press needle treatments
Dermal needle treatments

for a wide range of illnesses. There are also chapters on electronic acupuncture, and special moxa treatments.

Owing to the ambiguities and uncertainties, many students reach a 'plateau' and adopt one of two attitudes. They may concentrate solely on the practical application of 'symptomatic' acupuncture; or they may immerse themselves totally in the study of ancient Chinese texts, to the exclusion of modern research. Neither approach has validity for the practitioner of an ancient art, within a sceptical modern society.

We believe that acupuncture, although several thousands of years old, is still in its infancy, or perhaps in an uncertain adolescence. It is just entering the realms of microbiology, DNA, electromagnetic theory and laser beam technology. It is struggling towards scientific adulthood.

Our health depends on the functioning of our cells. These are constantly subjected to internal and external influences. One definition of physical life is 'Perpetually variable energy caused by exchanges between the organism and the external medium'. It is the function of acupuncture to maintain the health and efficiency of the cells by controlling the variable energy. Acupuncture achieves this by influencing the body's fourth circulatory system, which carries a form of electrical energy which the Chinese comprehend as ch'i. (The other three circulatory systems carry blood, lymph, and nervous information.)

This fourth system appears to have three functions. Firstly, it forms a link between man and the environment of electromagnetic energy in which he lives. Secondly, it controls the internal distribution of energy from its supply to its consumption. The third function is the supply of information to and from the cells. Thus the acupuncture points have the capacity for exchanging information between the surface of the skin, and the related organs, and ultimately with the nuclei of the cells.

This book is not an attempt to cover all aspects of acupuncture theory at an advanced level. We have taken two main aspects which we feel are most important and, at this stage, most illuminated by recent research. The book is written for the advanced student and the practising acupuncturist. It presumes that the reader is already familiar with the basic theory of Chinese medicine.

The following check-list may be useful. It gives the acupuncture subjects of which knowledge is presumed:
    Superficial paths of the 12 main meridians
    Superficial paths of Governor Vessel and Vessel of
        Conception
    Location of acupuncture points on the above meridians
    Pulse diagnosis
    Five-element theory
    Concept of *Yin* and *Yang*
    Circulation of energy in main meridians
    Chinese clock
    Treatments based on five-element theory
    Common symptomatic treatments
    Needle techniques

We have tried to avoid the use of Chinese terms when the same concept can be expressed easily in English. Similarly we have avoided Latin medical terms where common non-medical terms could be used.

1

The Creation of Ch'i

We have chosen only a small part from a very large area of theoretical knowledge for inclusion in this book. This is the part which seeks to explain the way in which man transforms and utilizes the energy available to him from outside.

The practising acupuncturist aims to effect changes in the way the energy is distributed and utilized throughout the body. He must also understand where and how the body energy is 'manufactured'. This knowledge can enable him to revitalize certain aspects of bodily functioning with the aim of ensuring that the food and air taken into the body are efficiently transformed into *ch'i*.

If the body is not performing this function efficiently, the system can turn inwards upon itself and deplete the body's reserves of basic energy. From all viewpoints this is unhealthy. From the viewpoint of the individual patient it leaves him less able to cope with future illnesses, or future situations which require energy if he is to survive. In time such depletion can lead to the inability to cope with even the normal demands of life. From a wider viewpoint it can weaken the essential energy which he inherited at birth, his *Yuan ch'i*. From a cosmological viewpoint, the patient is no longer operating as part of a universal system and is not 'in tune' with the basic life force around him. In terms of western medicine, such patients are often seen as 'constitutional inadequates'. Their pattern of recurring illnesses and failures is familiar enough, and it is usually accompanied by a lack of interest in life and a weakening of sexual capacity.

This chapter describes the 'Three-Heater' system when it is working efficiently. This efficient working presumes that the 'raw materials' taken into the body are of good quality. The patient's diet, his life-style and well-being complement any acupuncture treatment. They are therefore the concern of the acupuncturist, although beyond the scope of this book.

Ch'i, the life force, the vital energy, has many, many forms. One form evolves from another, and each has a specific application. Dr Manfred Porkert[1] gives nine shades of meaning to the word *ch'i*, and describes no less than thirty-two forms of *ch'i*, while stating that the list might easily have been longer.

One fact is clear. The word *ch'i* comes very close to our word 'energy'. It is always a definite form of energy, with a determined direction, or quality, or function, or purpose. The forms of *ch'i* mentioned in this chapter are:

Chen ch'i	True or nourishing energy
Cheng ch'i	Energy stored in the kidneys
Ching ch'i	Energy circulating in meridians
Hsien-t'ien ch'i	Inherited ancestral energy
Ku ch'i	Physiological energy from food
Tsung ch'i	Lung energy
Wei ch'i	Defensive energy of body
Yuan ch'i	The active part of *Hsien-t'ien ch'i*

also mentioned are:

Blood	Loose English translation of *Hsueh*, refers mainly to energy
Chin-yeh	Pure or essential body fluid
P'o and Hun	Conceptual aspects of *Shen*
Shen	Abstract or psychic energy

The creation of a living person from the wavelengths, frequencies, oscillations and potentials, which are the forms in which we conceptualize energy, must begin with this conception. Three forms of energy must come together to create human life. Two of these also have a physical presence, as the male sperm and the female ovum. The third intervening force is the cosmic, universal life force which may translate from Chinese as 'The Spirit of Heaven'.

The *ch'i* of the sperm and ovum is *Hsien-t'ien*, or 'ancestral' *ch'i*. The Chinese understood this form of hereditary energy thousands of years before modern biologists established the molecular structure of the double helix. They understood that the hereditary factor was established at conception and had a major role in the health and life-span of the individual. *Hsien-t'ien*, which is stored in the kidneys, is acquired only at conception, and must last for the person's lifetime. It circulates internally and has a vital influence, directly or indirectly, on all other transformations, and utilizations, of *ch'i* within the body. Although *Hsien-t'ien* cannot be increased, it can be weakened excessively by the failure to live a reasonably sensible life, or by

[1] Dr M. Porkert, *The Theoretical Foundations of Chinese Medicine*, MIT Press.

inept therapy, and life is shortened accordingly.

The child is conceived and lives for nine months in its mother's womb. Its only *ch'i* is the *Hsien-t'ien* of its parents. This affects its development as a foetus by interaction with the other energies which come from its mother via the umbilical cord. As a foetus it has no need for the complex *ch'i*-conversion functions of the 'Three-Heater' system.

Problems arise if the foetus is forced to birth before this complex system is ready to operate independently. This may occur in some cases when the foetus is malformed. It can also happen when the mother's energy is depleted, or the natural flow of energy is impeded by the excessive use of drugs, or by an inappropriate diet, or activity. The growing practice of induced labour is not one which appeals to many acupuncturists.

The processes of the Three-Heater system are not activated until the new-born baby takes its first breath. The processes of physiology which will support him throughout his life then commence. From the protection of his mother's womb, the baby is exposed to the direct and indirect influences of cosmic energy. The indirect form of cosmic energy is food, which comes up from the earth to unite with the more direct form of cosmic energy in the form of oxygen. The most direct form of cosmic energy are the radiations, electromagnetic or otherwise, which permeate the universe itself.

The Production of Ch'i and Fluid

Figure 1 is a diagrammatic explanation of the functioning of the Three-Heater system.

The upper heater is formed of the heart and lungs. The middle heater is stomach and spleen, and the lower heater contains liver and kidney, small intestine and bladder.

Yuan ch'i is the activated and physically employed part of *Hsien ch'i*. It acts much in the manner of a catalyst. It circulates from the kidneys, mostly by the eight extra meridians, and is concerned with the transmutation of one form of *ch'i* to another. On the diagram, *Yuan ch'i*, which resides in the kidneys, is represented by a seed-like shape.

We can now examine closely the processes by which the food we eat and the air we breathe are converted into vital energy:

(1) Food, the product of cosmic energy upon the surface of the earth – the 'essence of the earth' is taken into the stomach.

(2) Here, the activity of *Yuan ch'i*, from the kidneys drives off

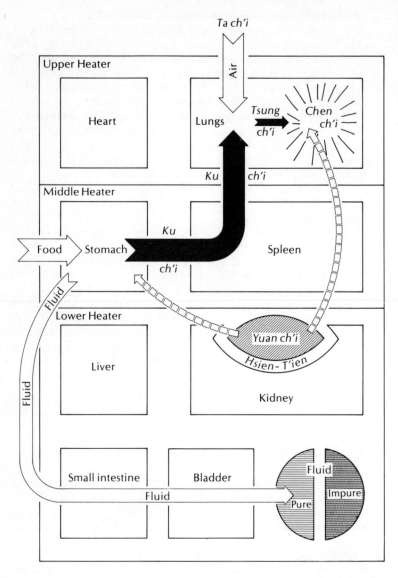

Figure 1
The Three-Heater System

the essential energy of food, called *Ku ch'i.*

(3) *Ku ch'i* goes to the spleen, which directs it to the lungs.

(4) In the lungs, the *Ku ch'i* combines with the energy of air, called *Ta ch'i.* This combined energy is called *Tsung ch'i.*

(5) This is still not the final form of energy which provides a reservoir of nourishment for the whole body. The influence of *Yuan ch'i* is again necessary. This changes the *Tsung ch'i* into *Chen ch'i.* It is now ready for distribution to the body.

In addition to *ch'i,* the body requires fluid and blood. Body fluids need to be constantly replenished, and for this they depend upon a balanced intake of food and liquid. The Three-Heater system controls the transport, utilization and excretion of fluids. The organs primarily concerned are lungs, small intestine and bladder. If one of these organs malfunctions there occurs edema, thirst, facial flabbiness, etc.

The Circulation of Chen Ch'i and Fluid

Figure 2 shows fluid separating from solids in the stomach, passing through the small intestine and bladder, to be further separated into pure and impure fluids.

Fluid and *Chen ch'i* circulate together through the five *yin* organs in the sequence of the *shen* cycle. *Chen ch'i* moves from the lungs to the kidneys, the liver, the heart and the spleen.

Fluid follows the same route, but starts from the kidneys. Each organ has its corresponding fluid. In the kidneys it produces parotid serus; in the liver it produces tears; in the heart it provides sweat; in the lungs it is mucous; and in the spleen it produces saliva (see Figure 2).

In diagnosis this knowledge can alert the acupuncturist to the location of the disease, when considered with other factors (see Chapter Five). The fluids, when produced in their appropriate amounts, serve as protectors and lubricants of the body. When they are deficient, or in excess, they are useful diagnostic indicators.

For example, mucous is part of the protection of delicate tissues. Some patients with chronic hay fever are prone to dryness of the nose which leads to even greater irritation by dust and pollen. In turn, this irritation and the resultant histamine reaction leads to the over-production of mucous. A little vaseline or petroleum jelly can help in the period while waiting for the acupuncture treatment to take effect.

Part of the *Chen ch'i* which circulates from the lungs, is retained by each *Yin* organ for its own use; some is converted

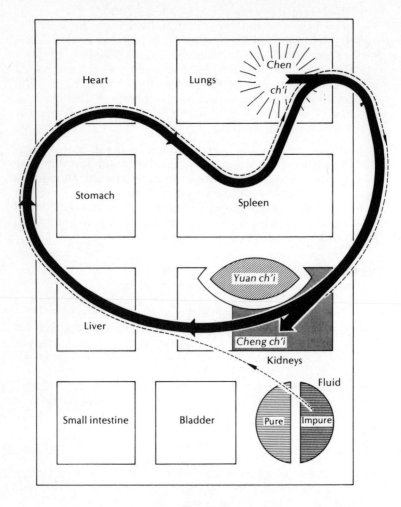

Figure 2
The circulation of *Chen ch'i* and fluid in the five *Yin* organs

to other forms of *ch'i*, and the balance is stored in the kidneys where it is called *Cheng ch'i*. This *Cheng ch'i* is a reservoir of refined, concentrated energy which is available when the body needs it. Traumatic injury, sudden emergencies and dangers summon up this reserve of energy. It is a similar concept to the 'Fight or flight' adrenotropic hormone which produces instant energy to fight or to run away.

Cheng ch'i is stored and consumed throughout the year. More energy is stored away in the *Yin* seasons of autumn and winter, than in the *Yang* seasons of spring and summer. This is in accord with the normal pattern of nature. If energy is wasted unnecessarily during the winter, there will be a deficiency later when it is needed in the spring to repulse the 'wind' diseases of spring. Thus the person's life may be shortened.

The state of a person's *Cheng ch'i* can be observed in his eyes, when viewed from the side. A sparkling, clear animated eye indicates that the person has ample stocks of *Cheng ch'i*. On the other hand, a cloudy, lack-lustre eye suggests a patient who may easily succumb to sudden infections.

Hsien-t'ien chi, the inborn constitutional *ch'i*, is stored within the kidneys. If this *ch'i* is depleted, all other kidney functions are affected. One effect is the weakening of the bones, which become soft. The bending of the softened long bones is common in very old people.

We have already stated that a small part of the *Chen ch'i* which circulates from the lungs through the *Yin* organs, is retained by each organ for its own use. Each organ may use *Chen ch'i* in three ways:

(1) Some *Chen ch'i* provides energy for the functioning of the organ (*Yin*).
(2) Some *Chen ch'i* is transformed into *Ching ch'i* in which form it circulates in the meridian system (*Yin/Yang*).
(3) Some *Chen ch'i* is transformed into *Wei ch'i* for the external defences of the body (*Yang*).

The remaining *Chen ch'i* continues the circulation of *ch'i* within the 5-element system (see Figure 3).

The *Yin* organs do not convert *Chen ch'i* into *Ching ch'i* and *Wei ch'i* in equal quantities. There is no general agreement about the exact details of the process. Dr Felix Mann, for instance, indicates that *Wei ch'i* is produced only in the lungs. A differing view is that *Wei ch'i* is produced mainly in the lungs, but that other organs may produce it to a lesser degree. The spleen produces a great amount of *Ching ch'i* much of which is used in the production of blood.

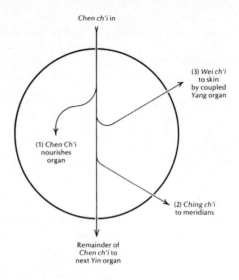

Figure 3
Functions of *Chen ch'i*

Wei ch'i is the defence energy of the body. Unlike *Ching ch'i*, which circulates only in the meridians, *Wei ch'i* is contained not only in the meridians, but also between the skin and muscles, in the fatty tissues of the abdomen and thorax, and in numerous capillary-like muscle/tendon meridians. *Wei ch'i* defends the body against external sources of illness. It accomplishes this by:

(1) Warming the skin.
(2) Causing perspiration.
(3) Nourishing the tissues.
(4) Controlling the opening and closing of the pores of the skin.

When *Wei ch'i* is circulating effectively, the skin is soft and the muscles and tendons are resilient to external influences. The electrical resistance of the skin is relatively low.[1]

The Nature and Formation of Blood
The exact sense in which the ancient Chinese doctors used the

---

[1] Research into Biofeedback demonstrates that the electrical skin resistance is lowest when the person is active and alert. The resistance increases as the person relaxes.

word 'blood' seems to defy precise definition in western terms. It is described as a 'radical', i.e., having the properties of energy more than of matter. Nevertheless, it is a definite substance which cannot be regarded as containing its own specific energy in manner of organs and tissues. This is because blood is constantly changing in volume and composition as new blood is introduced into the system.

Blood, like *Wei ch'i* and *Ching ch'i*, is manufactured within the Three-Heater system. It is formed by the interaction of *Ching ch'i* from the spleen, and pure fluid, which is known as *Chin-Yeh*. The blood circulates in the body and meridians (see Figure 4).

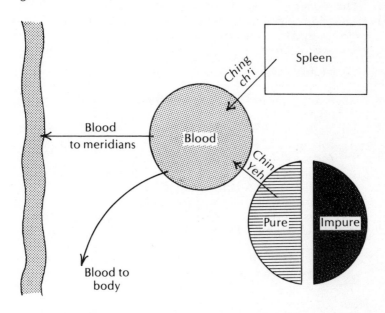

Figure 4

Other Body Fluids

The pure fluid of *Chin-Yeh* is the body's lubricant. *Chin-Yeh* is a composite word, of which *Chin* is the active *Yang* component, and *Yeh* is *Yin*.

Chin-Yeh moves in the meridians with the *Ching ch'i* and blood. It passes through the body tissues. *Chin* lubricates and nourishes the skin and the flesh. When it becomes externalized, under the control of the heart, it becomes sweat. *Yeh* is more internal in its action, lubricating the joints and tendons, protecting the brain, and filling the spine.

Summary

The three levels of circulation are:

For External Protection and Lubrication	For Internal Protection and Meridians	In the Internal Organs
1. *Wei ch'i* 2. *Chin* fluid	1. *Ching ch'i* 2. *Yeh* fluid 3. Blood	1. *Chen ch'i* 2. Impure fluid

The foregoing is by no means the only interpretation of the production and circulation of energy, blood and fluid. Most authorities, however they may differ on details, have the following in common:

(1) Nourishing *ch'i*, blood and refined fluid move in the meridians.
(2) Protecting *ch'i* and refined fluid move in the external tissues.
(3) Ancestral *ch'i*, or '*ch'i* of original heaven' is present at conception, resides below the navel or in the kidneys, and continues to influence a person's life.
(4) Surplus energy is stored in the kidneys, and is available on demand from the rest of the body.
(5) Nourishing *ch'i* is formed from food, water and air in the lungs, by the action of the middle and upper heaters.
(6) Blood, formed from *ch'i* and fluid, is partly or mainly energy.
(7) Refined fluid is formed in the lower heater from food and water, and is the lubricant of the body.

Shen

Ancient texts refer to *Shen* as a more abstract concept than *ch'i*. *Ch'i* is energy in action, or energy with a purpose. *Shen* a more speculative concept of 'pure' or perhaps 'guiding' energy which cannot be perceived directly.

Writers may refer to it as the guiding spirit which resides in the heart, analogous to a central government. Four functions are attributed to it, one for each of the other *Yin* organs:

(1) The *p'o function*, which directs the lungs, and the physical energy of *Ching ch'i*, *Wei ch'i* and blood.
(2) The *hun function*, which concerns the liver and directs all psychic and many mental processes, both conscious and unconscious.

(3) A *spleen function*, which is sometimes considered to control the processes of memory.

(4) A *kidney function*, which directs the process of will.

In effect, the *Shen* functions can not be directly known or controlled. They constitute the spiritual aspects of mankind, which determine his deeds, and his attitudes to others.

2

The Distribution of Ch'i

In Chapter One we looked at the functioning of the Three-Heater System and how it transformed, through various stages, external energy into *ch'i*, blood and fluid.

In this chapter we will follow the progress of this internal energy through the body. The components of the internal energy are:

Chen ch'i	Basic nourishing energy
Ching ch'i	The energy available for circulation in the meridians
Wei ch'i	Defensive Yang energy, not confined to the meridians
Blood	Consisting mainly of energy
Fluid	Perspiration, lubrication, and protection
Cheng ch'i	Reserve energy stored in kidneys

The circulation of the *Chen ch'i* within the *Yin* organs is described in Chapter One. *Ching ch'i*, *Cheng ch'i* and *Wei ch'i* are offshoots of *Chen ch'i*. They provide *Yin* and *Yang* energy to the body in the following manner.

Yin Energy

The principal source of *Yin* energy is the lung – heart – pericardium combination. *Yin* energy from these organs enters the Main meridians of the respective organs at chest level. The other *Yin* organs, kidney, liver and spleen, do not introduce *Yin* energy into the meridian system. On the contrary, they receive energy from their respective meridians at groin level (see Figure 5).

Yang Energy

Yang energy is supplied by the small intestine, colon and Three-Heater complex to their respective Main meridians at shoulder level. This *Yang* energy, derived from *Chen Ch'i* in the *Yin* organs, passes first to the coupled *Yang* organ, and thence to the *Yang* meridian.

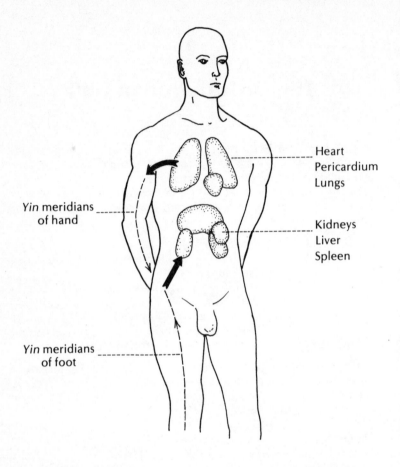

Figure 5
Energy exchange between the *Yin* organs and *Yin* meridians

Additional *Yang* energy, generated from *Chen ch'i* in the liver and spleen, and passed to gall bladder and stomach, is introduced into the gall bladder and stomach meridians at shoulder level. The bladder supplies energy from the kidney to the bladder meridian at groin level. This supplementary *Yang* energy has the constant function of bolstering the dwindling energy of the long *Yang* meridians of the foot.

The *ch'i* component of the *Yang* energy in the meridians comprises both *Ching ch'i* and *Wei ch'i*. The *Yang* energy is utilized by every part of the body. However, one region is of special importance. This is the region of the eye. The *Yang* meridians of the hand ascend to the orbit of the eye, and part of their energy goes to the brain. The remainder of the energy provides the initial energy for the *Yang* meridians of the foot, bladder, gall bladder and stomach (see Figure 6).

Kidney Energy

The kidneys have a key role in the production, storage, and circulation of *ch'i*. *Yuan ch'i* is stored in the kidneys. Its vital part in the conversion of external energy into *ch'i* is explained in Chapter One.

Cheng ch'i, the reserve energy of the body, is stored in the kidneys. This energy is available on demand. It can be summoned by the nervous system in an emergency. It is also available to the skilled acupuncturist within his patient.

In an emergency, the brain perceives danger. The normal reaction to fear is 'fight or flight'. Whether the person remains and defends himself or tries to escape, additional energy is needed quickly. This applies whether the danger is real or imaginary, physical or mental. *Cheng ch'i* provides this energy almost instantaneously. It is primarily a *Yang* response, and massive amounts of energy pass from kidneys to bladder and the bladder meridian (the need to urinate when confronted with danger is one aspect of the surge of *Yang* energy to the bladder).

The kidneys also distribute energy when it is needed, whether in an emergency or not, in two other ways. The first way is in accordance with the 5-element theory to the other *Yin* organs. The second way is through three of the extra meridians, *Jenmo*, *Dumo*, and *Chungmo*, which have their power sources in the kidneys. These are described in Chapter Four.

Variations in Meridian Energy

The nature of the energy being transported by the meridian system is far from being a smooth unvarying flow, even when

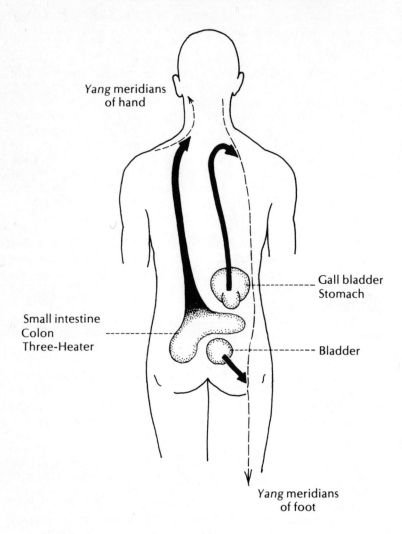

Figure 6
Energy exchange between the *Yang* organs and *Yang* meridians

the body is functioning perfectly and the pulses are balanced. There are four principal variations:

(1) The *Yin–Yang* balance.
(2) Changes in potential, i.e., there is more total energy available at certain places, and at certain times.
(3) Changes in the proportion of energy in the form of *ch'i*, as compared with blood or fluid.
(4) The balance of *Ching ch'i* and *Wei ch'i*.

Two factors influence the energy flowing in a healthy, fully-functioning body.

(1) The bodily functions themselves.
(2) The time of day, of the month, and of the year.

The Yin-Yang Balance
Of all terms used in acupuncture theory, *Yin/Yang* has proved the most difficult to express in one simple word or phrase. In different contexts in ancient texts it can have a very precise meaning (in the definition appropriate to law) or a very broad usage (to refer to complementary roles of male and female in society[1]). To overcome this, many books list opposite qualities as the only real attempt at both definition and explanation.

Our objection to these lists is not to the qualities or parameters chosen. The terms have been used so widely that almost any parameter can be seen in terms of *Yin* and *Yang* polarities. In many cases, however, such lists do not advance understanding of the *complementary* nature of the interacting forces. Instead, they emphasize the oppositeness and create a false impression that there is a dichotomy. There is no such dichotomy, only a general principle of a basic 'positive' and 'negative' of life. Even the use of these terms creates difficulties, in that popular usage implies that 'positive' means active, and 'negative' means inactive.

Another difficulty is that many such lists confuse general definitions with lists of Correspondences. Porkert clearly defines the two, and includes the following in his example:

[1] Dr M. Porkert, *The Theoretical Foundations of Chinese Medicine*, Chapter One.

	Definitions	Correspondences
YIN	Completion Condensation Conservative Responsive	Moon Coolness The right side The inside
YANG	Incipience Development Demanding Aggressive	Sun Heat The left side The outside

There has been a tendency in instructional materials to generalize very widely and to use the terms as if they were expression of two different forces, rather than aspects of the one force Yin/Yang. It is rarely correct to use Yin and Yang as separate nouns. They are *qualifying* terms, and both descriptive of activity of a different and complementary nature.[1]

LUNG	(LU)	Strong Yin	Increasing
COLON	(CO)	Normal Yang	
STOMACH	(ST)	Normal Yang	Decreasing
SPLEEN	(SP)	Strong Yin	
HEART	(HT)	Feeble Yin	Increasing
SMALL INTESTINE	(SI)	Strong Yin	
BLADDER	(BL)	Strong Yang	Decreasing
KIDNEY	(KI)	Feeble Yin	
PERICARDIUM	(PC)	Normal Yin	Increasing
THREE-HEATER	(TH)	Feeble Yang	
GALL BLADDER	(GB)	Feeble Yang	Decreasing
LIVER	(LI)	Normal Yin	

The *Nei Ching*, as often translated, gives the following intensities of Yin and Yang in the meridians, and indicates

[1] If Yin and Yang energy is considered in terms of electrical energy, it is usual to think of one as positive and the other negative. This makes the change-over from a Yin meridian (meaning more Yin than Yang) to a Yang meridian (more Yang than Yin) impossible to imagine.

Our own supposition is that Yang is analogous to high frequency and Yin to a lower frequency. We may then draw a simple scale from zero (no life) to Yin/Yang, on which 'more Yin' means a lower frequency, and 'more Yang' means a higher frequency.

whether the energy is increasing or decreasing. All the meridians of the hand are given as increasing, and those of the foot as decreasing. No mention is made of the level of *Yin* in the *Yang* meridians, or vice versa.

Graphs are sometimes drawn, based on this information, but they reveal no more about the changes in the strength of *Yin* and *Yang* than can be deduced from the table above.

The twelve Main meridians represent three circuits of the body, in which the energy varies as follows:

Circuit	Meridians	Yin	Yang
1	Lung, colon, stomach, spleen	Strong	Weak
2	Heart, small intestine, bladder, kidney	Weak	Strong
3	Pericardium, Three-Heater, gall bladder, liver	Average (increasing)	Weak

Apart from informing us which organs and meridians are strongly *Yin* or *Yang*, the above table is of value in helping us to decide when a treatment is most likely to be effective.

Changes in Potential and the Chinese Clock
Each meridian is at its maximum potential, i.e., has the greatest amount of available energy at certain times of the day or night. When a meridian is at its maximum potential it is at its highest level of *Yin* or *Yang*.

The timing of maximum *Yin*, therefore, is during the time when the circuit 1 meridians are at maximum potential, which is the eight-hour period from 3 a.m. to 11 a.m. Maximum *Yang* is during the time when the circuit 2 meridians are at maximum potential, which is the eight-hour period between 11 a.m. and 7 p.m. The period between 7 p.m. and 3 a.m., when circuit 3 meridians are at maximum potential, is one of weak *Yang*, but increasing *Yin* (see Figure 7).

The general principle of all acupuncture treatments is to assist natural energy movement. It is better, therefore, to treat a weakened patient when his *Yang* energies are increasing so as to strengthen this increase. Consider the graph of Figure 7. *Yang* is increasing between 9 a.m. and 1 p.m. and this is the best time to treat this type of patient.

Conversely, if the object is to drain excess energy, especially nervous energy, and to sedate the patient, this is more easily achieved between 5 p.m. and 9 p.m.

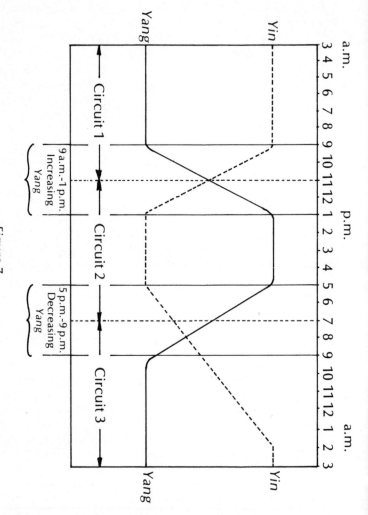

Figure 7
24 hour variations in Yin/Yang potential

The Balance of Blood and Ch'i

In Chapter One, blood is described as being mainly energy, but energy combined with physical substance, as distinct from *ch'i* which is pure energy. In some meridians the blood form of energy predominates and bleeding these meridians is an effective way of draining excess energy. The *Nei Ching* gives the following proportions of blood and *ch'i* in the meridians:

		Blood	*Ching Ch'i*
Strong *Yang*	(BL and SI)	Very high	Normal
Normal *Yang*	(CO and ST)	High	Very high
Feeble *Yang*	(TH and GB)	Normal	High
Strong *Yin*	(LU and SP)	Normal	Very high
Normal *Yin*	(PC and LI)	Very high	Normal
Feeble *Yin*	(HT and KI)	Normal	Very high

The only meridians where the blood energy content is high compared with the *ch'i* are: *bladder, small intestine, pericardium* and *liver*. These, and only these, meridians should be bled, by pricking with a triangular needle, or cupping. Only one or two drops of blood are necessary. If bleeding is in excess of this tiny amount it should be inhibited by pressure with a small pad of cotton wool. Bleeding should be avoided for a few days before and after the full moon.

The Balance of Ching Ch'i and Wei Ch'i

Wei ch'i, which is produced mainly in the lungs, is *Yang*. In all meridians the *Wei ch'i* is strongest at the most distal point, i.e., at the ends of the fingers and toes. This is the point of entry of the muscle/tendon meridian (see Chapter Three).

The predominance of *Wei ch'i* diminishes towards the wrist and ankle, from which areas the *Ching ch'i* continues to be the stronger.

There is also an annual variation of the depth of the *Ching ch'i* below the skin. The *Nei Ching* says that *Ching ch'i* begins to arrive in the meridians in springtime, and by the autumn it fills the meridians. In the autumn it begins to submerge, and in the winter is deep within the body.

In practice this means that the 'target area' is larger in summer than in winter. It should be borne in mind that the acupuncture point is not really on the surface of the skin, but some distance below the surface. In winter, when the *Ching ch'i* has withdrawn inwards, needling must be deeper and more precise. In the autumn and spring, the depth is medium. During the summer, the 'cross-section' of the meridian is

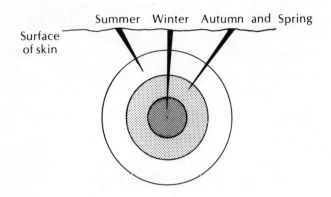

Figure 8
Cross section of a meridian (seasonal variations of energy)

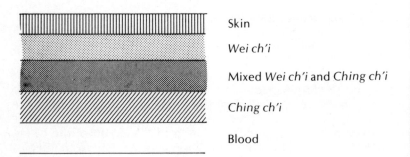

Figure 9
Energetic layers

greatly increased, so needling may be less deep, and the margin for error is greater.

The diagram in Figure 8 should not be taken to imply that meridians are channels with fixed banks. Dr Guido Fisch, at an international symposium on acupuncture, gave the meridian the form shown in Figure 9. Here the different forms of energy are shown in layers, one melting into the next.

The balance of *Ching ch'i* and *Wei ch'i* is also affected by day and night. During the day, almost all *Wei ch'i* flows in the muscles and tendons, and the network of tiny meridians which serve them (see Chapter Three). At night, part of this *Wei ch'i* flows internally, and any treatment to increase *Yang* energy is less likely to be successful at night.

3

The Complete Meridian System

The complete meridian system, by which we mean all the pathways of energy between the surface of the body, and the organs, muscles and all other parts of the body, is uncharted. By the levels of contemporary understanding it is too complex to comprehend. Every part of the body appears to be represented in the ears, in the eyes, and probably on the hands and the soles of the feet. If we are to postulate 'meridians' connecting these points we are faced with a network of communications beyond imagination.

Future research into the mechanisms of acupuncture may well lead to the conclusion that the concept of meridians or pathways is not necessary to explain the apparent transfer of energy from one set of body cells to another. In this respect, the body possibly resembles the brain, and indeed why should it do otherwise? The brain may appear to function rather like an immense telephone exchange, but all research indicates that such is not the case. It functions by some quite different, but not yet understood, process.

Meanwhile, the traditional concept of meridians is the only viable hypothesis. Most importantly, it is clinically effective.

The 71 Important Meridians
These are as follows:

12	Main meridians	
2	Extra meridians, *Jenmo* and *Dumo* with their own acupuncture points	The 8 Extra Meridians
6	Extra meridians without discrete points	
14	*Lo*, or linking meridians, from 12 Main meridians, *Jenmo* and *Dumo*.	The 15 Lo Meridians
1	Great *Lo* meridian of the Spleen	
12	Connecting meridians, joining each pair of main meridians, *Yin* and *Yang*, at the extremities	
12	Divergent meridians from Main meridians	
12	Muscle/Tendon meridians from *Ching* point of each Main meridian	
71	TOTAL	

The 12 Main Meridians

The Chinese term is *ching-mo* meaning 'energetic conduits'. Dr Porkert suggests the full sense is 'to guide the rhythmic manifestations of energy along definite conduits' or 'network of energetic conduits'.

The superficial paths of the main meridians, and the location of the acupuncture points upon these paths, are described in detail by almost any book on acupuncture.

The meridians do not terminate at the most proximal acupuncture point, although they may appear to do so on most charts. There are important internal connections from these points to the *Yin* and *Yang* organs, and sometimes to other meridians.

The most important connection from the most proximal point on each meridian is to the organ which bears the same name as the meridian. The second most influential connection is with the coupled organ.

Meridian	*First Internal Connection*	*Second Internal Connection*	*Other Connections*
Heart	HT	Small intestine	Spleen and lung meridians
Small intestine	SI	Heart	
Bladder	BL	Kidney	Brain
Kidney	KI	Bladder	
Pericardium	PC	Three-Heater	
Three-Heater	TH	Pericardium	
Gall bladder	GB	Liver	
Liver	LI	Gall bladder	Kidney meridian
Lungs	LU	Colon	Liver and kidney meridians
Colon	CO	Lungs	
Stomach	ST	Spleen	Lung, liver and small intestine
Spleen	SP	Stomach	

The 8 Extra Meridians

These are the subject of Chapter Four.

The 15 Lo Meridians

The 12 *Lo* meridians, or *Lomo*, which connect with the 12 Main meridians, join these meridians at the *Lo* Points. From each *Lo* point , there are two branches of the *Lo* meridian. The connecting meridians also start from the *Lo* points.

The first branches of the *Lo* meridians extend the influence of Main meridians to various parts of the body. Their routes are irregular:

Meridian	Lo Point	Pathway of Lo Meridian
Heart	HT 5	Adjacent to the Main heart meridian; then up through the chest and throat to the root of the tongue; then to the tissues behind the ball of the eye
Small intestine	SI 7	Along the arm to the shoulder joint
Bladder	BL 58	Ascends leg to abdomen to join *Lomo* of *Dumo*, and connect with bladder
Kidney	KI 4	Upwards adjacent to the Main kidney meridian to the region below the pericardium; then to the lumbar region
Pericardium	PC 6	Adjacent to the pericardium; Main meridian to the region of pericardium
Three-Heater	TH 5	Along the arm to enter the chest
Gall Bladder	GB 37	Down the leg to the dorsum of the foot
Liver	LI 5	Upwards along the tibia to the testicles and penis in the male, to genital organs in the female
Lungs	LU 7	To the palm of the hand, spreading along the thenar eminence
Colon	CO 6	Up the arm and over the shoulder and neck to the angle of the jaw; then enters at an angle to the root of the teeth
Stomach	ST 40	Up the lateral edge of the tibia, through the abdomen and chest to the throat
Spleen	SP 4	Up the leg to intestines and stomach

There are at least three schools of thought about the paths, and the functions, of the second branch of the *Lo* meridians. These are:

(1) That each *Lo* meridian links with the *Lo* meridian, of the coupled Main meridian. For example, the heart *Lo* meridian joins the small intestine *Lo* meridian. This is perhaps a simplistic view which confuses the *Lo* meridians with the connecting meridians (see below).

(2) That each *Lo* meridian links with the paired Main meridian. The same comment applies as to (1).

(3) A much more interesting idea was put forward by Mr Van Buren when lecturing in Australia. He suggested that the *Lo* meridians constitute a reservoir of energy between the Main meridian and its specific organ. This would be capable of absorbing excess energy from the Main meridian, and provide an energic 'buffer' or safety-valve. This excess energy might be absorbed by the organ itself, or be tapped by needling the *Lo* point, and passed on to the coupled meridian by the connecting meridian, which also starts at the *Lo* point.

Dr Porkert describes the *Lo* meridians as being delicate branches of the Main meridians, which supplement the functions of the Main meridians.

The two extra meridians, *Jenmo* and *Dumo*, also have *Lo* meridians. The *Lo* point of *Jenmo* is VC 15, below the Xiphoid process. From this point the *Lo* meridian spreads through the abdominal region. The *Lo* point of *Dumo* is GV 1. From here (a point with strong *Yang* energy) the *Lo* meridian ascends on each side of the spinal column to the back of the neck; then it spreads over the upper region of the head; then turns and descends down both sides of the scapula to join the *Lo* meridian of the bladder. It terminates in the lumbar region.

The 15th *Lo* meridian, called the Great *Lomo* of the Spleen, branches off the Main Spleen meridian at SP 21. It spreads over the sides of the rib cage in the region of the pectoris lateralis. It is considered to be in control of all other *Lo* meridians. The control point SP 21 is sometimes listed as a point in general use by mainland Chinese acupuncturists, but, in practice, points with more specific effects are usually preferred.

The 12 Connecting Meridians
These are the meridians which provide a 'cross-over network' at the region of the wrist and hand, or ankle and foot, between coupled meridians, one *Yin* and the other *Yang*.

The connecting meridians carry the energy from one

meridian to the next. In the process the energy is converted from being primarily *Yin* to primarily *Yang*, or vice versa. This is not a sudden process, but one which takes place progressively within the hand and wrist, or within the foot and ankle.

The point on the leg or arm at which this transformation and transference starts, or finishes, is the *Lo* point. At this point the Connecting meridian leaves the Main meridian and spreads out into a network of small channels which connect with the coupled meridian. Small channels, all part of the Connecting meridian, leaves the main meridian between the *Lo* point and the *Ching* point (the most distal point) of the Main meridian. The change of polarity, from *Yin* to *Yang* or from *Yang* to *Yin*, occurs within these small channels.

After losing energy at the *Lo* point, the Main meridian loses some of its polarity, *Yin* or *Yang*. As further energy leaves the meridian, the polarity continues to decrease until, at the *Ching* point, the effective polarity is slight. Only a comparatively small amount of low polarity energy passes from one *Ching* point to the *Ching* point of the coupled meridian.

As an example, the heart meridian is *Yin*. At the *Lo* point, which is HT 5, some of the *Yin* energy is diverted into the Connecting meridian. By the rule that 'There is always *Yin* within *Yang*, and *Yang* within *Yin*', the balance of *Yin* and *Yang* is altered. There is now less *Yin* to the same quantity of *Yang*. At the Source Point, HT 7, there is even less *Yin* and the same quantity of *Yang*. At the *Ching* point, HT 9, there is only slightly more *Yin* than *Yang*.

The 'gathering point' for the energy of the Connecting meridians is the Source Point of the coupled meridian. The Source Points are, HT 7, SI 4, BL 64, KI 3, PC 6, TH 4, GB 40, LI 3, LU 9, CO 4, ST 42 and SP 3.

The 12 Divergent Meridians

In the *Nei Ching*, the physician Chi-Po tells the Emperor that the understanding of these meridians distinguishes the skilled physician from the unskilled. They may be considered of equal importance to the Main meridians.

The *Yang* divergent meridians leave their Main meridians on the limbs, and rejoin them at the head or shoulders. The *Yin* divergent meridians, however, leave their Main meridians at various points, but do not rejoin them. Instead (with the exception of TH) they join the coupled *Yang* meridian, of the same element.

It is only on account of the Divergent meridians that the three *Yin* meridians of the foot, kidney, liver and spleen can be used effectively for conditions which involve the head. The

Main meridians themselves do not ascend above the trunk. The Divergent meridians are internal, have no acupuncture points, and have important connections with the organs of the body.

The pathways of the Divergent meridians can best be described in pairs:

Heart and Small Intestine (Figure 10)

The Divergent meridian of small intestine (a) leaves the main meridian distal to SI 9, penetrates the axilla to (b) the heart and (c) the small intestine. It ascends to join the Divergent meridian of heart (d) at BL 1. BL 1 is the terminal point of the extended small intestine meridian.

The Divergent meridian of heart diverges (e) from the main meridian internally (below GB 22, under the axilla). It passes through the throat and face to join the Divergent meridian of small intestine at BL 1.

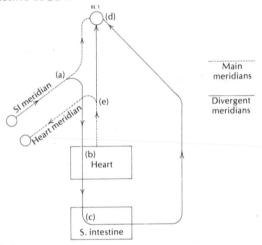

Figure 10
Divergent meridians: heart and small intestine

Kidney and Bladder (Figure 11)

The bladder Divergent meridian leaves the Main bladder meridian between BL 55 and BL 54 (a). It continues with the Main meridian to the point *Yinshang*[1] (b) from which point a branch goes to the anus and gall bladder (c). The principal section of the Divergent meridian ascends each side of the spinal column (d) and branches out to the kidneys (e) and the

---

[1] *Yinshang* is 2 *tsun* proximal to BL 51. It is a non-meridian point.

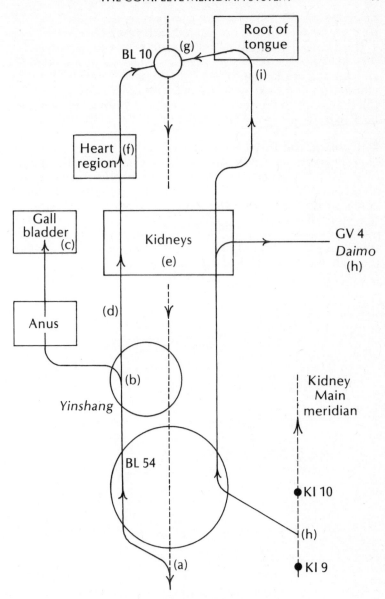

Figure 11
Divergent meridians: kidney and bladder

heart region (f). From here it emerges in the muscles at the back of the neck to join the Main Bladder meridian at BL 10 (g).

The kidney Divergent meridian starts between KI 9 and KI 10 (h). It connects with the bladder Main and the bladder Divergent meridians at BL 54 (a). From here it travels up to the kidneys (e) and links with the extra meridian, *Daimo*, at GV 4 (h). It ascends to the root of the tongue (i) from whence it goes back to unite with the Main bladder meridian at BL 10 (g).

Pericardium and Three-Heater (Figure 12)
The Divergent meridian of the Three-Heater has the special function of connecting the brain with the Three-Heater meridian, and the organs of the Three-Heater system. It makes contact with – or passes through – the brain. Contact with the Main meridian is in the region of TH 17, behind the ear (a). This is also the entry point to the brain. From here, the Divergent meridian passes through the Three-Heater system (b), ascends through the supraclavicular fossa and over the head to the vertex, GV 20 (c).

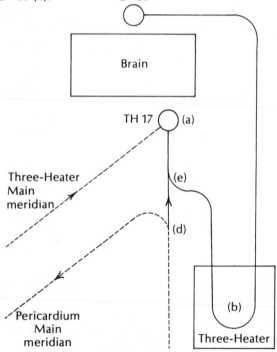

Figure 12
Divergent meridians: pericardium and Three-Heater

The pericardium Divergent meridian diverges from the Main meridian about 3 *tsun* below the centre of the axilla (d). It penetrates the chest and links with the Divergent Three-Heater meridian (e) with which it ascends round the throat to join the Main Three-Heater meridian in the region of TH 17 (a).

Gall Bladder and Liver (Figure 13)

The gall bladder Divergent meridian leaves the Main meridian at GB 30 (a). It skirts the hip joint and enters the pubic hair region to be joined by the liver Divergent meridian (b). The combined Divergent meridians ascend and spread out within the rib cage, passing through the gall bladder and liver (c). It then has some contact with the heart (d), ascends to the side of the larynx, runs laterally across the cheek and jaw to enter the face and reunite with the Main gall bladder meridian at GB 1 (e).

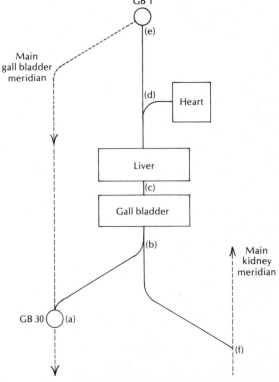

Figure 13
Divergent meridians: gall bladder and liver

The liver Divergent meridian diverts in the region of LI 4, on the dorsum of the foot (f) and ascends the leg to meet the gall bladder Divergent meridian in the region of the pubic hair (b).

Lung and Colon (Figure 14)
The lung Divergent meridian leaves the internal Main lung meridian about 3 *tsun* below the axilla (a). The principal branch ascends through the supraclavicular fossa and along the throat to join the Main colon meridian at the face (b). A subsidiary branch of the lung Divergent meridian descends to the colon and meets the colon Divergent meridian (c).

The Divergent meridian of colon diverts at CO 15 (d) to enter the spinal column at GV 14 (e). It then descends to the colon and meets the lung Divergent meridian (c).

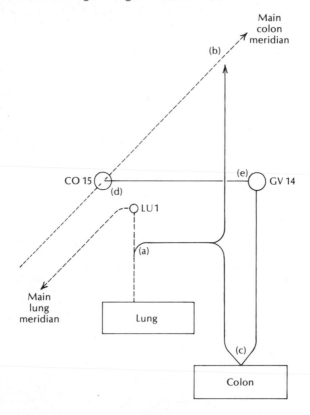

Figure 14
Divergent meridians: lung and colon

Stomach and Spleen (Figure 15)
The stomach Divergent meridian leaves the Main meridian at
ST 32 (a) and ascends towards the great trochanter where it
enters the internal abdominal region and the stomach (b). It
then enters the spleen (c) and makes some contact with the
heart (d). The meridian then travels upwards along the throat
into the mouth. It emerges on the surface of the face and
rejoins the stomach Main meridian at ST 1 (e).

The path of the spleen Divergent meridian is short but
important. It diverts at the point *Chihsia*[1] (f) and joins the
stomach Divergent meridian in the upper part of the thigh (g).

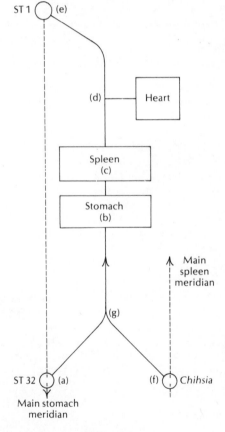

Figure 15
Divergent meridians: stomach and spleen

[1] *Chihsia* is a non-meridian point 2 *tsun* below SP 11.

The 12 Muscle/Tendon Meridians

All muscle/tendon meridians start at the *Ching* point of the Main meridian. This is the most distal point of the meridian. Generally speaking, each muscle/tendon meridian accompanies the Main meridian throughout its length, and terminates by joining other muscle/tendon meridians as follows:

Muscle/Tendon Meridians	Meeting Place
Yin meridians of the hand, heart, pericardium and lungs	The chest
Yang meridians of the hand, small intestine, Three-Heater, colon	The side of the head, in front of the ears
Yin meridians of the foot, kidney, liver and spleen	The genitals
Yang meridians of the foot, bladder, gall bladder and stomach	The cheek

The muscle/tendon meridians should not be thought of as clearly-defined conduits, but rather as a vast network of branches and capillaries which radiate from the *Ching* points through the skin and over the muscles and joints.

The muscle/tendon meridians carry only *Yang* energy. This includes *Ching ch'i*, and *Wei ch'i*. The *Ching ch'i* nourishes the muscles and joints, and the *Wei ch'i* defends the body from external sources of disease.

The effect of needling the *Ching* point depends upon the energy state of the Main meridian.

(1) If the *Yang* energy in the coupled Main meridians is low, needling the *Ching* point will summon energy from the muscle/tendon meridian.
(2) If energy is needed in the areas served by the muscle/tendon meridian, and there is *Yang* energy to spare in the Main meridians, this can be diverted into the muscle/tendon meridian.

The Total Meridian System

Figure 16 gives a simplified impression of the meridians attached to a pair of coupled Main meridians, *Yin* and *Yang*, of the same element. It is not intended to be an accurate representation of any particular pair of meridians. It illustrates:

(1) The two *Main meridians*, with internal connections to the organs at one end, and an undefined link between the distal *Ching* points at the other end.
(2) *Connecting meridians*, transforming *Yin* into *Yang*, or vice versa. Although a network, the effective connection is from the *Lo* points to the opposite Source points.
(3) *Lo meridians* which take a variety of routes, different for each meridian.
(4) *Divergent meridians*, also with irregular routes. Both *Yin* and *Yang* Divergent meridians join the *Yang* Main meridian.
(5) *Muscle/tendon meridians* which radiate from the *Ching* points through the skin and over joints and muscles.

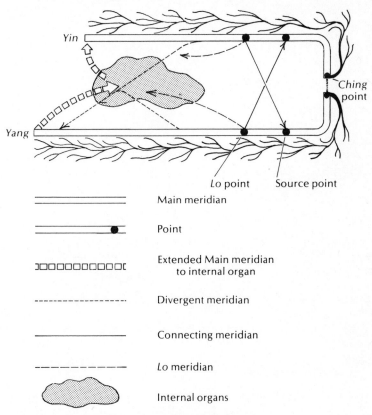

Figure 16
The total meridian system

4

The Eight Extra Meridians

Chinese tradition gives us remarkably little detailed information about the clinical use of the eight extra meridians. The pathways are described, as is the manner in which they are paired and the points which control them.

Modern Chinese practice often appears to ignore them, but many western acupuncturists would testify that extra-meridian treatments are exceptionally effective.

One theory about the functioning of the extra meridians describes them as a system which distributes *Yuan ch'i*. Another, in modern Chinese publications, describes the extra meridians as having the role of regulating the *ch'i* and blood in the 12 Main meridians. These may amount to much the same thing. *Yuan ch'i*, which is stored in the kidneys, and kidney energy in general are regarded as catalysts or motivating forces for the rest of body. By controlling the distribution of kidney energy, the eight extra meridians would effectively regulate the energy in the other meridians. But this is not necessarily the only function of the extra meridians.

In addition to its effect upon the meridian system, *Yuan ch'i* is necessary for five other body functions which are not specifically mentioned in ancient Chinese texts. These are:

(1) The circulatory system
(2) The blood, and blood-cell manufacturing process
(3) The brain and nerves of the spinal column
(4) The uterus, or male genital organs
(5) The biliary system

These functions, too, come under the influence of the extra meridian system.

Only *Jenmo* and *Dumo* (Vessel of Conception and Governor Vessel) have their own acupuncture points. The other six extra meridians share acupuncture points with the Main meridians. *Jenmo*, *Dumo* and *Chungmo*, all of which originate in the lower abdomen, particularly the kidneys, are considered especially important.

Jenmo

The Vessel of Conception is usually shown as starting in the pelvic cavity. It emerges at VC 1 on the perineum from whence it runs centrally up the front of the body to VC 24, which is in the depression below the lower lip. From here it divides and runs bilaterally round the mouth to ST 4, crosses under the nose and extends to ST 1.

At the mouth, *Jenmo* does not become continuous with *Dumo*, as it may appear. Both meridians enter the mouth and descend internally to the pelvic region. One theory holds that *Jenmo* and *Dumo* form a continuous loop in the form of a figure-8. The energy changes from *Yin* to *Yang*, and back again. By this theory, *Jenmo* emerges from the anus and is almost totally *Yin*. It ascends to the mouth where it is about equally *Yin* and *Yang*. As it descends internally it becomes increasingly *Yang* until it emerges as *Dumo*, almost totally *Yang*. Then, as *Dumo* it ascends and becomes more *Yin*. At the mouth it is equally balanced *Yin* and *Yang*. It descends internally,

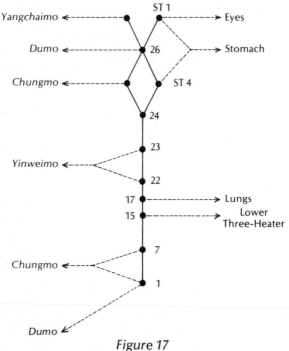

Figure 17
Connections with *Jenmo*

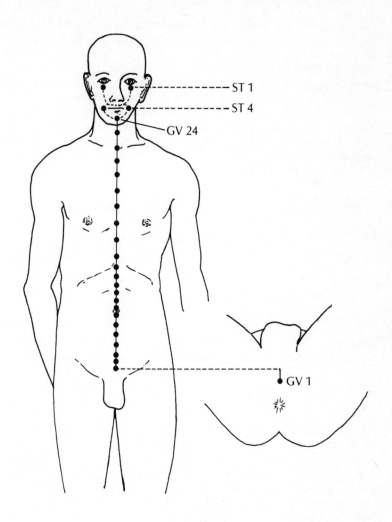

Figure 18
Extension to *Jenmo*

becoming increasingly *Yin* until it emerges from the anus as *Jenmo*.

Jenmo is the 'sea' of all *Yin* meridians, with which it has indirect connections. It connects with the eyes at ST 1, with the stomach at ST 4, with the lower Three-Heater at VC 15, with the lungs at VC 17.

The lower points are urogenital; the middle points are digestive, and the upper points are thoracic. Deficient energy is often indicated by skin itching. Excess energy is indicated by painful abdominal skin. *Jenmo* controls pregnancy and menstruation. It is indicated, preferably with *Yinchaimo*, for all female insufficiency problems.

Other indications are:

Asthma	Hernia
Bronchitis	Head and neck pains
Coughs	Hayfever
Difficult breathing	Influenza
Dyspepsia	Laryngitis
Epilepsy (with *Yinweimo*)	Mouth diseases
Eczema	Pneumonia
Eye problems	Pharyngitis
	Urogenital problems

Dumo

Dumo emerges from the pelvic cavity at the perineum. GV 1 is at the tip of the coccyx. It ascends along the middle of the spinal column and communicates with the kidney at the lumbar region. It ascends to the vertex, communicating with all other organs on the way. It enters the brain, descends to the upper lip and penetrates the mouth to GV 28. It makes contact with *Jenmo*.

Some authorities give the origin of *Dumo* in the *Yang* kidney, from whence it passes through the genital organs to VC 1. The main energy then proceeds to GV 1 and *Dumo*, and the remainder, moves forwards to VC 2. At this point it divides into two muscle/tendon meridians, of which the anterior branch goes to the muscles of the heart and spleen, and the posterior branch goes to the bladder muscle/tendon meridian at the back.

Figure 20 shows another version of the *Dumo* connections. The coupling with *Taimo* at GV 4 is speculative, but, without it *Taimo* would be the only extra meridian unconnected with the whole extra-meridian network. The origin of *Dumo* is shown as the right (fire, or *Yang*) kidney. An important *Lo* meridian of *Dumo* is shown starting from GV 1, ascending the spine, and

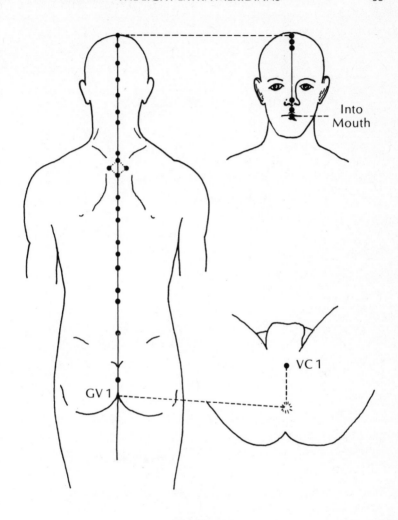

Into
Mouth

VC 1

GV 1

Figure 19
Dumo

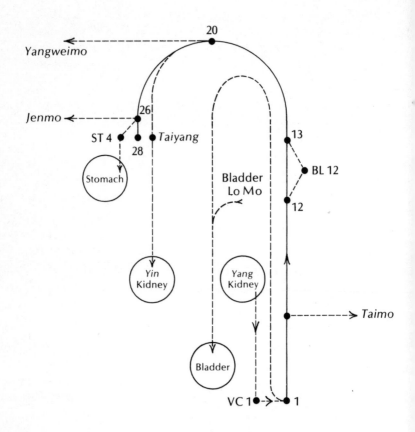

Figure 20
Connections of *Dumo*

the back of the head almost to the vertex, then descending to join the bladder *Lo* meridian going to the bladder.

The non-meridian point *Taiyang*[1] is a potent point on account of its position on the extension of *Daimo* from the head to the left (water, or *Yin*) kidney.

Dumo connects with the stomach by way of ST 4, and has a link with *Jenmo* at GV 26. All the individual points of *Dumo* which are level with the *Shu* (AEP) points on the bladder meridian, have connections with the corresponding organs. Bladder and kidney are also affected by GV 2, 3, 4 and 5. There is an additional connection with BL 12 from GV 12 and GV 13. This, together with BL 38, is the 'cancer' point.

Dumo is indicated for:

Conjunctivitis	Neck Pains
Frontal neuralgia	Phlegmy cough
Febrile diseases	Running eyes
Haemorrhoids	Urine retention
Hernia	Sterility
Lumbago	

When *Dumo* is overactive the indications are headaches and pain in the eyes caused by excess *Yuan* and *Ching ch'i*. The spine may also become stiff. When *Dumo* is chronically deficient in energy the patient tends to be round-shouldered and feel heavy-headed.

Chungmo

Chungmo originates in the pelvic cavity, especially the kidneys. It emerges from the groin at VC 1. The next point along the sulcus is at ST 30. *Chungmo* then joins the kidney meridian from KI 11 to KI 21. There is a connection from KI 15 to VC 7. From KI 21 it ascends bilaterally to the larynx, and terminates in a network round the mouth. A bilateral branch is sometimes presumed down the legs, posterior to the medial malleolus to SP 4 and the dorsal part of the foot.

It is sometimes considered that the true kidney points KI 11 to KI 21 are very deep below the surface of the skin and have no meridian connections of their own, but only a connection to the surface and *Chungmo*. Even this academic speculation serves to emphasize the importance of *Chungmo* in the distribution of kidney energy.

Chungmo influences the eyes, probably by the bladder Separate meridian into which the kidney Separate meridian

---

[1] *Taiyang*. In the depression, about one *tsun* lateral to the external canthus. Often called the sun point. Dr Felix Mann gives it as XH 3.

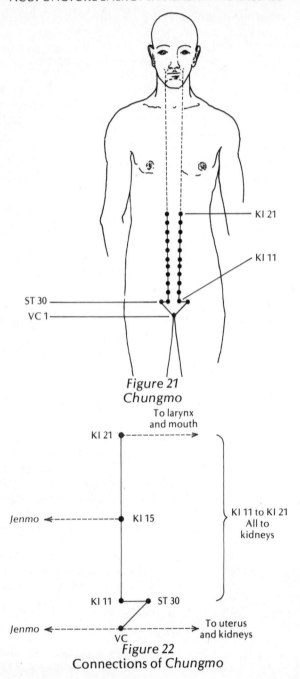

Figure 21
Chungmo

Figure 22
Connections of *Chungmo*

flows, carrying kidney *Yang* energy to BL 1. *Chungmo* is also indicated for:

Digestive ulcers	Lumbago
Gastric ulcers	Palpitations
Hyperacidity	Stomach ache
Gynaecological disorders	Heart diseases

and all organic diseases in which there is an hereditary factor. *Chungmo* is described as 'The sea of blood' and 'The sea of 12 meridians'.

Taimo

Taimo originates in the floating ribs and surrounds the body like a belt. It is considered to equalize the energy of all the meridians which pass the middle of the trunk. Traditionally, its acupuncture points are LI 13, GB 26, 27 and 28. Current opinion often adds GV 4, and a connection to GB 15. The latter is a point on *Yangweimo* (coupled with *Taimo*) and one of the contact points with the brain.

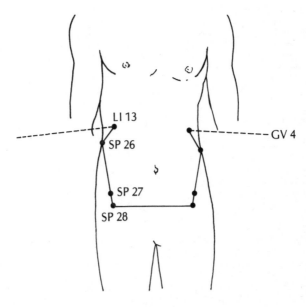

Figure 23
Taimo

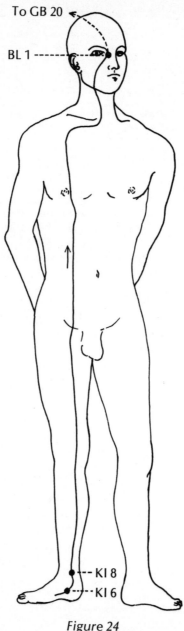

Figure 24
Yinchaimo

Taimo is not used frequently, except in conjunction with *Yangweimo*.

Yinchaiomo

Yinchaiomo, or the *Yin* heel vessel, has its origin in the region of KI 2 or KI 6, according to which authority we accept. It ascends the leg, and passes through all the *Yin* organs of the body to region of ST 12, then through the throat to BL 1. Some sources believe that it continues over the skull to GB 20 and enters the brain.

Yinchaiomo and *Yangchaiomo* meet at BL 1, and perhaps go together to GB 20. When a person is healthy the energy in the two extra meridians is balanced. They are both concerned with transporting *Yuan ch'i*. Weak ankles sometimes indicate that the energy in these two meridians is seriously unbalanced.

The only points on *Yinchaiomo* are KI 6, K 8, BL 1 and possibly GB 20. It is treated mainly for organic problems in women, especially fluid retention. Main indications are:

Sexual weakness	Lack of sexual pleasure
Difficult childbirth	Toxic pregnancy
Cystitis	Post-partum pains and bleeding
Constipation	Bladder weakness
Motor impairment in legs	Hypersomnia

Yangchaiomo

Yangchaiomo starts in the region of the external malleolus and has three bladder points, BL 62, 61 and 59. It ascends over flanks to GB 29, then winds round the shoulder to SI 10, CO 15 and 16. Then to the face, ST 4, 3 and 1, and the inner canthus of the eye at BL 1. From BL 1 it goes over the head to GB 20.

Yangchaiomo is traditionally only used when treating males. It may be used for female patients with care, but they should always be seen again within a few days in case of side-effects.

It has a hormonal action, including the stimulation of the production of adrenocorticotropic hormone (ACTH). Production of this is more beneficial to the patient than treatment by synthetic corticosteroids. These have notorious, sometimes eventually fatal, side-effects such as increased blood-pressure, depression, peptic ulcers, weakened bones, susceptibility to infection, and increased weight due to salt retention.

Yangchaiomo may therefore be used to treat any of the conditions for which western medicine prescribes cortisone. These include asthma, giant hives, rheumatic conditions, and to suppress inflammation. It may be noted here that 'curing'

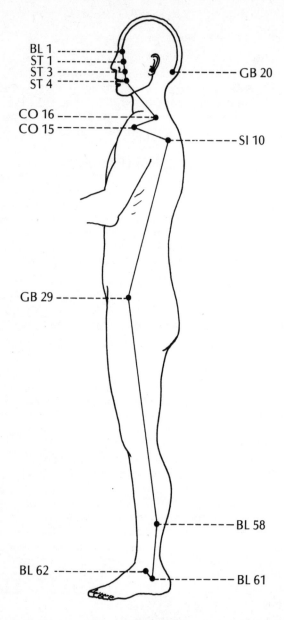

Figure 25
Yangchaimo

inflammation by chemo-therapy is not necessarily beneficial to the body. For example, in the case of an inflammatory reaction to an allergy, the stimulation of additional ACTH to reduce the inflammation is beneficial. However, when swelling and inflammation is caused by the plasma containing anti-bodies to infection, this should not be suppressed. It is part of a natural healing process.

Other indications for *Yangchaiomo* include:

Locomotion and articulation problems, lumbago, rheumatism, etc.
Hormonal inbalances (use BL 1 and 6, in addition)
Obsessions, manic depressive states, paranoia, insomnia (use ST 3 and 4, GB 20, in addition)
Spasms, epilepsy, etc. (sedate BL 62)

Yinweimo

This originates in the *Yin* meridians of the foot, but the first superficial point is KI 9. It ascends inside the leg to the groin and up the trunk to LI 14, SP 13, 15 and 16. From these four points there are connections by the vagus nerve system to all *Yin* organs, especially the heart. It terminates at VC 22 and 23.

Yinweimo is used traditionally to treat all cold, meaning energy-deficient, conditions. *Yangweimo*, on the other hand, is used for treating hot conditions. When *Yinweimo* is diseased the patient may have heart pains even though the heart itself is not diseased. This is caused by the blood, which is supplied by the spleen by the intervention of the kidneys, being supplied in incorrect amounts. When *Yinweimo* is seriously deficient in energy, the genitals are painful. *Yinweimo* is indicated for:

Emotional instability   Cardiac pain
Timidity   Indigestion
Nervous laughter   Abdominal pains, ulcers
Anxiety and apprehension   Pain in pit of stomach
Amnesia   Constipation
Nightmares   Varicose veins

Yangweimo

Yangweimo starts below the lateral malleolus at BL 63. It ascends the outside of the leg to GB 35, then up the body to SI 10. There is a branch to GB 24. The shoulder points are SI 10, TH 15 and GB 21. *Yangweimo* then ascends the neck and cheek to the following sequence of points: ST 8, GB 13, GB 14, GB 15, GB 16, GB 17, GB 18, GB 19, GB 20, GV 16 and GV 15.

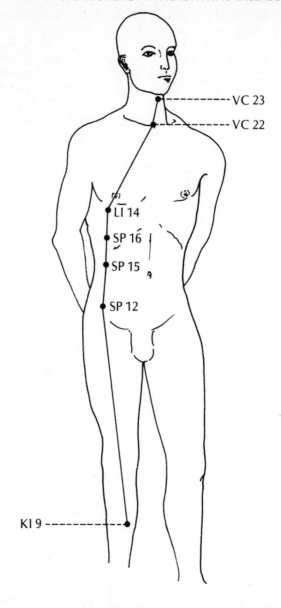

Figure 26
Yinweimo

This is by no means the only version. Dr Felix Mann[1] shows the meridian as going first to the back of the head and coming forward to terminate at GB 13. He includes GB 24 as being on the meridian. Dr Porkert[2] gives the same route, without GB 24. In the *Outline of Chinese Acupuncture*[3] the route is the same as shown in illustration 28, excluding GB 24.[4]

Yangweimo has strong links with the brain. It strongly affects the gall bladder and bladder meridians. These are the outermost and second outermost protective levels against external illness-producing energy. *Yangweimo* therefore has a strong protective function. It carries *Yuan Ch'i*, in its *Yang* form, to support the external protection of *Wei ch'i*.

When *Yangweimo* is diseased or lacking in energy, the patient feels cold, is prone to infection from external evils, and suffers from colds and chills. *Yangweimo* is also indicated for:

Acne
Arthritis of toes and
    fingers
Boils
Earache
Thinness
Tinnitis

Mouth abscesses
Mumps
Nose bleeding
Swollen neck
Toothache
General weakness

[1] Dr Felix Mann, *The Meridians of Acupuncture*.
[2] Dr Manfred Porkert, *The Theoretical Foundations of Chinese Medicine*.
[3] Published by Foreign Languages Press, Peking 1975.
[4] The authors also offer a tentative theory that *Yinchaiomo* and *Yangchaiomo* form an energy circuit, energized by the *Yin* organs. This would convey *Yin* energy to the brain (which receives mainly *Yang* energy from the Main meridians) and return by way of the *Yang* organs to the legs. The sequence of points suggests that this is more probable than the accepted idea that both extra meridians are ascending.

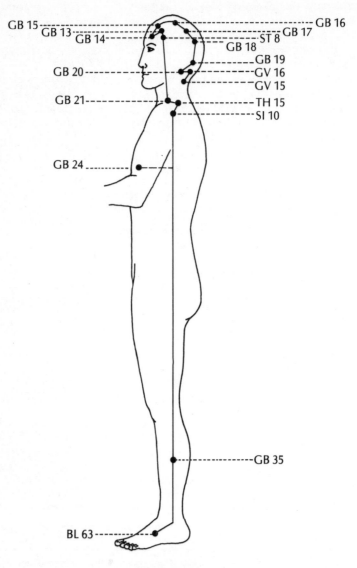

Figure 27
Yangweimo

The Eight Extra Meridians Used in Pairs

Treatments using the eight extra meridians are most effective when the meridians are used in pairs as follows:

Jenmo Yinchaimo }	controlled by	{ LU 7 KI 60
Dumo Yangchaimo }	controlled by	{ SI 3 BL 62
Chungmo Yinweimo }	controlled by	{ SP 4 PC 6
Taimo Yangweimo }	controlled by	{ GB 41 TH 5

Each extra meridian is controlled by a Master Point which may, or may not, be a point on the meridian.

The treatments are slightly complicated, and merit a careful stage-by-stage explanation:

Stage 1
If using *Jenmo* and *Yinchaiomo*, needle LU 7.
If using *Dumo* and *Yangchaiomo*, needle SI 3.
If using *Chungmo* and *Yinweimo*, needle SP 4.
If using *Taimo* and *Yangweimo*, needle GB 41.

(As an aid to memory, use the Master Point of the extra meridian with the *shorter* name.)

Stage 2
Needle this point *unilaterally*. On the left side for males, right side for females.

Stage 3
Now needle, unilaterally, the Master Point of the other meridian, on the *opposite side*.

Stage 4
Needle any additional points to be used. Leave the needles for 20 minutes, or as determined by the pulses. Remove the needles in the *reverse* order to that in which they were inserted.

Stage 5
Needle the Master Point of the second meridian, on the left side for males, right side for females.

Stage 6
Needle the Master Point of the first meridian on the opposite side. Leave the needles for half the period of the first pair of needles. Remove in the reverse order.

Jenmo and Yinchaiomo   Use LU 7 and KI 6
For organic female problems, especially involving water metabolism and hormone imbalance at menopause.

When edema occurs in a woman at menopause, there is an excess of gonadotropic hormone, associated with a deficiency of female sex hormones. *Yinchaiomo* has a strong connection with BL 1, which is the point that controls the pituitary gland. This is a small gland which pours into the bloodstream an incredible variety of secretions which control our bodily functions, and without which we could not survive more than a few days. The hormones controlled by the pituitary gland include the growth hormone, ACTH, gonadotropic hormones, lactogenic hormones and thyrotropic hormones. The pituitary gland, through the hypothalamus, affects our emotions and the autonomic nervous system.

ACTH, or adrenocorticotropic hormone, influences the adrenal glands, which produce epinephrine. This controls blood pressure, pulse, respiration and blood sugar content. It relaxes the bronchial muscles, and it is the trigger for the alarm-reaction in an emergency, which releases the reserves of *ch'i* stored in the kidneys. ACTH is also involved with asthma, giant hives, and rheumatoid arthritis.

KI 6, the Master Point of *Yinchaiomo*, influences the suprarenal gland. Additional points which may be introduced at Stage 4 are:

KI 8 for additional influence on the suprarenal gland
BL 1 to stimulate the pituitary gland
VC 9 for all water problems
KI 18 and BL 1 for menopausal hot flushes

Dumo and Yangchaiomo   Use SI 3 and BL 62
For locomotive and articulation problems including rheumatism, lumbago, etc., mostly in male patients. Some acupuncturists claim that it is essential to use BL 1 and BL 60 to achieve effective hormonal balance. This seems to be an overstatement, for good can be obtained without BL 1, use of which may impose a strain on the patient (not to mention the acupuncturist). Other additional points which may be introduced at Stage 4 are:

BL 59, BL 61 for rheumatism in the legs
SI 10, CO 15, CO 16 rheumatism in arms and shoulders
ST 3, ST 4, GB 20 rheumatism in the back
GV 12, GV 20 for nervous conditions
Chiachi points between GV 12 and BL 12 for multiple sclerosis

Chungmo and Yinweimo   Use SP 4 and PC 6

This pair of extra meridians is specially indicated when the patient has organic deficiency attributable to heredity. *Chungmo* closely allied to the kidney meridian, and the kidney, in which is stored the *Yuan ch'i.*

Yinweimo has a double action. Through VC 22 it is related to the entire nervous system. *Chungmo* and *Yinweimo* are indicated for heart insufficiencies, and to improve the blood supply from the liver and spleen. Points which may usefully be needled at Stage 4 are those which are tender on palpation, thus indicating organic illness. These are:

KI 11 to KI 21
SP 13 to SP 16
LI 14
VC 22, for thyroid conditions

Taimo and Yangweimo   Use GB 41 and TH 5

Taimo's liver and gall bladder points are valuable for headaches, migraine and genital troubles. LI 13 influences the liver's capacity to neutralize unemployed sex hormones.

Additional points which may be needled at stage 4, but only if painful under pressure, are:
LI 13
GB 26, GB 27, GB 28

Balancing Pulses with the Eight Extra Meridians

When the state of the energy in the meridians, as shown by the pulses, is unbalanced, the acupuncturist may attempt to achieve a harmonious distribution of *ch'i* by application of the principle of the 5-elements. This is often effective, though not always so.

There is an alternative which does not involve the 5-element principle. In certain cases it is possible to achieve the desired results, quickly and easily by use of the extra meridians. This is not surprising considering that the balancing of energy throughout the body is one of the major functions of the eight extra meridians.

We may consider an extra meridian as influencing the energy

supply in any meridian with which it is connected. The greater the number of points of contact, the greater the effect on that meridian. For example the gall bladder meridian is influenced by four of the eight extra meridians:

Taimo	at 3 points
Yinchaiomo	at 1 point
Yangchaiomo	at 2 points
Yangweimo	at 11 points

It is also indirectly affected by *Dumo*.

Obviously *Yangweimo* has the greatest effect on the gall bladder meridian. The following table shows the number of points of influence of the eight extra meridians.

	HT	SI	BL	KI	PC	TH	GB	LI	LU	CO	ST	SP
Jenmo				*				*			2	*
Dumo			1				*				*	
Chungmo				11							1	
Taimo							3	1				
Yinchaiomo			1	2			1					
Yangchaiomo			4				2			2	3	
Yinweimo				1				1				3
Yangweimo		1	1			1	11				1	

To 'balance pulses' using an extra meridian, the procedure is:

Stage One
Ascertain if there is one extra meridian which has points of influence, direct or indirect on *all* the meridians upon which an effect is desired. If there is no such extra meridian, apply the 5-element principle.

Stage Two
If an extra meridian is available, needle the Master Point, unilaterally, on the left side for men and on the right side for women.

Stage Three
Now needle the Coupled Point of the meridian on the opposite side. The 'Coupled meridian' is the Master Point of the paired meridian, i.e. LU 7 and KI 6; SI 3 and BL 62; SP 4 and PC 6; GB 41

* indicates strong indirect influence

and TH 5. Leave both needles until the pulse indicates that all possible improvement has been made.

Electronic Stimulation of Extra Meridians
This is normally effective using dense/dispersal frequencies (see Chapter Eight). Duration of treatment is approximately halved.

5

The Cause and Diagnosis of Disease

Before treatment, the acupuncturist should attempt to define, in terms of Chinese medicine, what is wrong with the patient. It is not necessarily sufficient to merely identify the symptoms in western terms, for example, by saying that the patient has a headache.

Chinese diagnosis is not as difficult as it may appear, as the task is made to seem more complex by the conflicting terms employed by different writers and different schools. For the purpose of this book, we have selected certain terms and applied them only to one clearly-defined condition each. *Yin* and *Yang*, for instance, have been restricted to the site of the disease, as distinct from the symptoms of the disease, or even the causes of the disease.

Every disease may be defined in five different categories:

	Yang	*Yin*
Location of disease in organ and/or meridian	*Yang*	*Yin*
Energy condition of symptoms	Hot	Cold
Energy condition of whole body	Full	Deficient
Source of disease	External	Internal
Duration of disease	Acute	Chronic

The terms *Yang* and *Yin* can be applied to all five categories, but to do so only creates unnecessary confusion. We will consider each of the five categories separately.

Yin and Yang
The first diagnostic consideration is the location of the disease. Is it only in or along the main meridian? Has it reached the organs? Which meridians or organs are affected?

Firstly, consider any abnormal conditions along the pathways of the meridians; for example, pain, swelling or skin eruptions. In some cases, the location of the symptom may not, in itself, be evidence as to which meridian is at fault. For instance, an ear infection may be due to a diseased meridian of small intestine, Three-heater, gall bladder or even kidney. Other symptoms, and the pulse diagnosis must be taken into account.

Generally speaking, diseases of the meridians are fairly easy for the observant acupuncturist to diagnose. The following are typical examples:

Gall Bladder and Liver Meridians
If either meridian is at fault, there will often be a 'greenness' about the patient. The eyes, nails and tendons are liable to be affected. There may be either emotional anger, or silence and a tendency to cry.

If the Gall bladder meridian is 'hot', i.e., having an excess of energy, we can expect headache, heaviness, pains in the side and ribs, and dizziness. The patient may have a bitter taste in his mouth and be easy to anger.

Kidney
With hot symptoms of the kidney meridian, the patient may easily have a full, swollen abdomen, or sweat a great deal. Conversely, cold symptoms of the same meridian include a cold, weak or sore body, and a weak sex drive.

Small Intestine
With hot symptoms, we can expect excessive sweating, a hot body and a congested chest perhaps with swollen jaws or pain along the SI meridian. The patient may be melancholic.

The above are examples of what the acupuncturist should be looking for. For a more detailed list of symptoms, see 'Energy condition of symptoms' in this chapter.

It is not usual for two meridians to be involved. The meridian first affected may quickly influence another meridian with which it has a special relationship. The common relationships are:

(1) With the *paired meridian*, of the same element. For example, when the spleen meridian is cold, perhaps because of bad diet or excessive exercise, the stomach meridian will often be found to be hot (meaning deficient, and excessive energy respectively). One meridian appears to have taken energy from the other.

Conversely, when the colon meridian is hot with perverse energy, i.e., infected, its partner meridian,

lungs, will gradually become colder and exhausted.
(2) With an *opposing meridian*. This is most often on the *Ko*-cycle, usually with the *Yin* meridians. For example, if the lung meridian is hot (metal element) the liver meridian may be affected and become cold (wood element).

Conversely, when the kidney meridian energy is cold, the heart meridian will 'burn' strongly.

When two meridians are involved, it is necessary to study the overall condition of the patient before deciding which meridian is the more important and should be treated first. Sometimes, of course, it is possible to treat both meridians simultaneously.

To summarize: the location of the disease may be at three levels. These are:

(1) In the meridians only. If only *Yang* meridians are involved, the condition is firmly *Yang*. If *Yin* meridians are involved the condition could be described as *Yin/Yang*. All meridian conditions are, to some degree *Yang*.
(2) If the disease has penetrated to the *Yang* organs it may be thought of as *Yang/Yin*. All diseases of internal organs are, to some extent, *Yin*.
(3) If the disease has reached the *Yin* organs, it is definitely a *Yin* disease.

Energy Condition of Symptoms
The Chinese use the term *Hsu* and *Shih*, sometimes to describe symptoms, and sometimes in a more general sense to describe the energy state of the body as a whole. To avoid confusion, we have adopted 'hot' for *Shih*, meaning being full, or having an excess, of energy. This applies only to symptoms. 'Cold' means *Hsu*, which is the state of being deficient in energy. Hot and cold do not necessarily refer to temperatures, although 'hot' symptoms are often associated with dry, painful, perspiring conditions, and 'cold' symptoms with pale, chilly, watery conditions.

Other 'hot' symptoms are inflammation, fever, blood congestion, constipation, stiffness, sharp pains, headaches, restlessness, etc.

Other 'cold' symptoms are often less obvious. They include weakness, excess fluid, diarrhoea, cramps, low body temperature, numbness and a general absence of correct functioning.

When related to various meridians, certain symptoms may be considered as typical:

Meridian	Hot Symptoms	Cold Symptoms
Heart	Insomnia Nightmares Thirst Excessive laughter	Coldness and pain in left shoulder and arm Cardialgia
Small Intestine	Deafness Tinnitis Swollen jaw Excessive sweating Dark urine Melancholia	Diarrhoea
Bladder	Lumbago Headache Painful eyes Spinal pain Blocked nose Hot, painful shoulders Stiff hips and knees	Heavy jowls Thickened neck Triple chin (also Spleen)
Kidney	Intestinal swelling Constipation Blurred vision Aneuria Abdomen swollen Excessive sweating Salty taste in mouth Nervousness	Hot dry mouth Lumbago Diarrhoea Cardialgia Swollen larynx Dry sore throat Cold limbs or feet Fatigue Fear Anxiety Excessive sleep No sex drive
Pericardium	Heart pains Palpitations Red complexion Flushed face	
Gall Bladder	Headaches Deafness Foggy vision Painful ribs and side Dizziness Bitter taste in mouth Restless sleep Pulse wiry and rapid Bad temper	Cold feet Insomnia Weakness in legs Inability to make decisions Timidity

Meridian	Hot Symptoms	Cold Symptoms
Liver	Genital disorders Bad temper	Fear Depression
Lungs	Abnormal perspiration Harsh breathing Chest congestion Panting Hard dry cough Fainting Frequent, scant urination Feeling chilly in hot weather Tongue dry and hard Urine dark Sore throat Excessive thirst Face red and fever Mental agitation	Shortness of breath Breathing difficulties Blocked nose Very white nose Phlegmy cough Excess phlegm Low energy Edema of whole body Edema of face, around eyes Tongue white and slippery Yawning Increased urination
Colon	Constipation Mouth hot and dry Urine dark and scanty Deafness Tooth decay Tongue yellow and dry Pulse rapid	Diarrhoea Abdomen painful and rumbling
Stomach	Frequent hunger caused by too-rapid digestion Abdomen hot Face burning Tender bleeding gums Abnormal perspiration Nose bleeding Swollen neck Tooth decay Bloody taste in mouth Bad smell in mouth Pain in legs Dry lips and mouth Yellow urine	Front of body cold Shivering Lips white Abdominal edema
Spleen	Stomach pains Constipation Acute pain round heart Whole body painful	Dysentry Loosening of articulation of whole body Mental depression

No symptoms are shown for the Three-Heater meridian, because the three areas of the body represented by this meridian are not necessarily in the same state. For example, a patient may have a 'hot' upper section, and a 'cold' lower section, or vice versa.

The Body State: Full or Deficient?

Before attempting to treat a patient, the conscientious practitioner will consider the patient's overall health. In commonsense terms, we must ask ourselves, 'Is the patient strong enough to withstand the treatment we have in mind?' This is especially important when we are faced with the problem of draining excess, but perverse, energy from an already-weakened patient.

The signs of fullness of energy are:

(1) A strong body
(2) A clear mind
(3) Clear eyes
(4) A healthy skin
(5) Most pulses well-defined
(6) A firm voice

The signs of a body deficient in energy are:

(1) Under-nourishment
(2) Muscles weak
(3) Depressed or confused mind
(4) Unhealthy-looking skin
(5) Weak or muddled pulses
(6) Thin or shaky voice
(7) Dull eyes

There are thus four combinations of energy states: hot or cold symptoms, in a full or deficient body:

(1) *Hot* symptoms, *full* body. The patient's health is generally good. Disease energy (infection, etc.) is combating the body energy. The pulse is usually floating, rapid, smooth, large or strong. The symptoms are typically pain, inflammation, etc.

(2) *Hot* symptoms, *deficient* body. The body energy is weak, and failing to counteract the energy of the disease. The pulse is floating, weak and small. Symptoms may include fever and inflammation.

(3) *Cold* symptoms, *full* body. The symptoms are not obvious; there is no inflammation or high temperature. The pulse is sunken but full, showing energy within the

body to fight the disease.

(4) *Cold* symptoms, *deficient* body. The illness is chronic. The pulse is sunken, small and weak.

If the body energy is full, a draining or sedating treatment presents no dangers. When the body energy is deficient, care must be taken not to drain away body energy in an attempt to drain disease energy. This sometimes becomes a necessary risk when treating an acute disease which is becoming worse each day.

The Source and Progress of Disease: External or Internal?
There are three sources of disease:

(1) *External*: these include climatic conditions, heat, cold, humidity, wind, dryness, etc., and physical injuries. These usually affect the *Yang* meridians and the illness is commonly hot and full.
(2) *Emotional*: when these cause internal damage it tends to be in the *Yin* organs.
(3) *Faulty diet*: The *Yin* energy may be weakened and unable to prevent external sources of disease penetrating the body.

The external, emotional and dietetic factors which cause disease are identified in the *Nei Ching*. The following table indicates which organ or meridian can be injured by each factor:

External cause of Disease	Emotional cause of Disease	Dietetic cause of Disease	Organs of this Element Will be Affected
Warmth Heat	Excessive joy Irresponsibility	Bitter flavours	Fire
Humidity Damp	Indecision Brooding	Too much sweetness	Earth
Arid dryness	Sadness Excessive mourning	Too much spicy food	Metal
Cold	Worry Fear	Too much salt	Water
Wind	Repressed anger	Sour food	Wood

Any consideration of the external or cosmic causes of disease must consider the Chinese descriptions of the pairs of meridians. These are:

{ Small Intestine Bladder	are	Greater *Yang*	
{ Gall Bladder Three Heater	are	Lesser *Yang*	The 3 Levels Of *Yang*
{ Colon Stomach	are	Sunlight *Yang*	
{ Spleen Lung	are	Greater *Yin*	
{ Pericardium Liver	are	Absolute *Yin*	The 3 Levels Of *Yin*
{ Heart Kidney	are	Lesser *Yin*	

Modern Chinese literature sometimes describes Greater *Yin* and Greater *Yang* as external gates; lesser *Yang* and absolute *Yin* as axis; and Sunlight *Yang* and Lesser *Yin*, as internal gates.

The outermost, and most vulnerable meridians, are small intestine and bladder. As a pair they form the longest meridian in the body. The bladder is most prone to attack in the winter, and the small intestine in summer.

The second most vulnerable meridians are gall bladder and Three-Heater. Of these the gall bladder meridian is the more vulnerable. It criss-crosses over the face and head and is especially vulnerable to the wind (element wood). The important point GB 16, in Chinese called *Fengfu* or 'the mansion of the wind', is the point at which the perverse energy of wind enters our systems and spreads to other meridians. When cold winds blow, and we huddle into our scarves, or turn-up our coat collars, it is GB 16 that we are protecting.

The third level, colon and stomach, is the least vulnerable to external attack, of the *Yang* meridians.

The fourth level is lung and spleen. This is the first of the *Yin* levels. Lung is the coupled meridian of colon, of the element metal. Spleen is the coupled meridian of stomach, of the element earth. The link between third and fourth levels is therefore strong.

The fifth level is pericardium and liver, and the innermost level is the vital organs heart and kidney.

Figure 28 shows the six levels diagrammatically. External, perverse, disease-causing energy attacks at the outer levels and progresses inwards, attacking from level to level. It progresses until it is brought to a halt by the defensive energy of the body. This defensive energy can be summoned by the acupuncturist who correctly interprets the symptoms and deduces the depth to which the disease has penetrated.

The condition may also be made worse by faulty treatment which can carry the disease to a deeper level. For example, in treating a disease which is only affecting the bladder meridian, the acupuncturist should be wary of any treatment which might take energy from the gall bladder meridian. To do so would be inviting the disease to move inwards to the weakened gall bladder meridian.

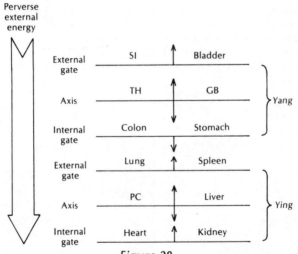

Figure 28
The level-by-level penetration of external energy

The success or otherwise of the acupuncture treatment may be indicated by the appearance of new symptoms. For example, a patient being treated for a chronic digestive problem develops symptoms which point to a 'hot' small intestine condition. This is a good sign for the disease is moving outwards from stomach-level to small intestine-level. If, on the following visit, the patient complains of headache and painful eyes which are both 'hot' bladder symptoms, the patient is well on the way to recovery.

As we have seen, externally-caused illness is usually first manifested on the *Yang* meridians, but this is not always the case. The *Yin* meridians may be attacked directly by cosmic energy. The arms and legs, where the skin is soft, are most vulnerable to the perverse energy of the wind and cold.

Although the *Yin* meridian is attacked, it is the *Yang* coupled organ which is first affected, and which repels the attack. Even if the disease reaches the *Yin* organs it will not be able to remain long enough to cause damage, unless the body is exceptionally deficient in energy. So, outside perverse energy such as wind and cold can not cause disease in the heart, liver, spleen, kidney or lungs of a healthy person.

So far, we have assumed that a disease has only one external cause, but this is an over-simplification. Sometimes two or more external factors are involved. A wind, for instance, is rarely just wind. It is more often, especially if it is harmful, a hot wind, or a dry wind, or a cold humid wind. In the latter case the cold may affect the bladder, the humidity may affect the stomach, and the wind itself may attack the gall bladder. The Shanghai College states that wind and cold attack the upper body, and damp attacks the lower body.

The location of pain is an aid to diagnosis of which meridian is diseased:

Location of Pain	Meridians Probably Concerned
Forehead	Small intestine Bladder
Side of head between ears and eyes	Three-Heater Gall bladder
Cheeks	Stomach Colon
Neck	Bladder
Chest, back pectoral muscles	Bladder Gall bladder Stomach

The Duration of the Disease: Chronic or Acute?
These terms are used as in western medicine. As we have seen, many diseases first affect the *Yang* meridians and organs, and eventually progress to the *Yin* organs. The body is not seriously damaged until the disease reaches the *Yin* organs and becomes chronic.

In general, acute conditions respond more readily to treatment than chronic conditions.

6

Symptomatic Treatments

Many books on acupuncture give useful lists of 'prescriptions' for various diseases. The books by Dr Felix Mann[1] and Dr Wu Wei Ping[2] are recommended. The treatments suggested in this chapter have been compiled without reference to these, or any other popular text books, in English. In many, but not in all cases, the treatments have been tried in our own practice.

Diseases are listed alphabetically. Five different treatments are given under each heading, according to the type of treatment. The five treatments are:

(1) *Main Points*: For normal needle acupuncture.
(2) *Ear Points*: Usually used in conjunction with main points. To be needled.
(3) *Needleless*: Points recommended when the electrode is taped to skin.
(4) *Press Needle*: Ear points in which a press-needle may be left between treatments.
(5) *Dermal*: Body points in which a dermal needle may be left implanted between treatments.

Under some headings, there is a sixth entry:

(6) *Moxa*: see Chapter Seven.

This draws attention to the fact that there is a special moxa treatment for the disease, which is explained in detail in the following chapter.

Main Points
The formulae given in this category are mostly those recommended in a variety of modern Chinese textbooks. Only the most-used points have been included.

It is not suggested that all points should be used in one treatment. Points should be selected (a) in accordance with

[1] Dr Felix Mann, *The Treatment of disease by acupuncture*, Heinemann.
[2] Dr Wu Wei Ping, *Chinese Acupuncture*.

established principles of point selection, near-and-distant points, etc. (See Wu Wei Ping and others) and (b) with consideration of the principles of 5-element theory and pulse diagnosis. One or more *additional* points may be added to the treatment.

All points referred to are on the standard Chinese charts.[1] The numbering of the bladder meridian points is the 'European' method, i.e. *Yinmen* is BL 51, *Weiyang* is BL 53, and *Weichung* is BL 54, etc. The kidney meridian loops round the medial malleolus with *Taihsi* as KI 3 (this differs from the numbering used by Dr Felix Mann). The stomach meridian starts below the eye at *Chengchi*, with *Touwei* as ST 8 at the top of the branch (some books use a different numbering).

The abbreviations used for the meridians are:

HT	heart
SI	small intestine
BL	bladder
KI	kidney
PC	pericardium
TH	Three-Heater
GB	gall bladder
LI	liver
LU	lung
CO	colon (large intestine)
ST	stomach
SP	spleen
VC	Vessel of Conception (*Jenmo*)
GV	Governor Vessel (*Dumo*)

Ear Points
These are in locations shown on sheet 2 of *The Newest Illustrations of Acupuncture Points*, with the addition of several new points on the back of the ear (see Figure 29).

Ear points may be divided into three types:

Type A	Points with an emotional or hormonal effect. e.g. *Shenmen*, subcortex.
Type B	Points which relate to a particular organ or part of the body. e.g. knee, stomach.
Type C	Points which affect a condition. e.g. cough or hunger.

As a general guide, not more than two, or perhaps three, ear points should be used during a single treatment. A typical

[1] *The Newest Illustrations of Acupuncture Points.*

treatment using ear points might be:

1 type A ear point
1 type B or C ear point $\Big\}$ unilateral

Several main body points
from series (1) formula $\Big\}$ bilateral

If electronic stimulation is applied to ear points not more than two needles should be in the ear at the same time, kept apart from each other by a small piece of cottonwool. The most suitable needles are $\frac{1}{2}$ inch fine-gauge Chinese needles.

The acupuncture points of the ear are very small, not more than about 1mm diameter and it is difficult to establish their exact locations. Not only do point locations vary from person to person, but in many cases the charts show only the area within which the point may be found. Often only the 'hot' or sensitive points can be identified with any degree of certainty. The task is made much easier with a good electronic point locator, although the active points are sensitive or actually painful when tested with a blunt probe. With the latter method, the area of the point is explored with uniform pressure and the patient is asked to report the location of any pain.

Needleless
The most usual form of needleless acupuncture using electronic stimulation consists of the taping (PVC insulation tape is convenient to use) the electrode to the skin instead of inserting a needle into the skin and clipping the terminal to the needle.

The normal type of electronic stimulator may be used. Special leads should be prepared with small metal discs, about $\frac{1}{4}$ inch diameter in place of the usual 'crocodile' clips. The end of each lead, any soldering, etc., should be insulated with nail varnish, so that only the small disc is in electrical contact with the skin.

Treatment should be longer than for electronically-stimulated needle treatment, and a higher voltage is required to overcome the increased resistance of the skin. Needleless electronic acupuncture can be effective, and it has obvious advantages for nervous or needle-phobic patients, and children.

Research in Hong Kong[1] suggests that better results are obtained from specially chosen 'needleless' acupuncture points than from the points which would have been used for

[1] The Chinese Medicine and Acupuncture Research Centre, Kowloon.

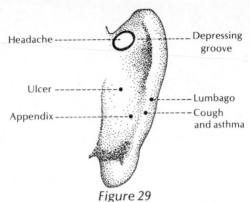

Figure 29
New acupuncture points at the back of the auricle

normal symptomatic needle treatments. The points are meridian points, and the choice of meridian is conventional. These points are given in the following symptomatic treatments.

Implant Points
Centuries ago, in China, the patient could be treated daily by the village doctor. Many acupuncture treatments are much more effective if treatment can be daily, especially for the first few treatments. In western urban conditions this is usually impossible to arrange. Any intervening treatments must be left to the patient himself, or be in the form of a needle or needles left implanted in the skin.

In some cases the patient can treat himself with moxa or acupressure. In other cases either (a) a press needle, or (b) a dermal needle, may be in position for up to a week, between treatments.

Under the heading 'Implant points' we give the press-needle points of the ear. This is the most popular form of on-going treatment. The needles have 2mm penetration, and a circular base. They resemble a tiny skeleton drawing-pin. One or more press-needles may be left in position for a week, protected by an adhesive dressing. A small clipping from the end of a piece of adhesive plaster is almost invisible and very suitable for the purpose.

As a general rule, type-A points have the greatest on-going effect. A type-B, or type-C may be added when appropriate. The points listed in the following symptomatic treatments should be considered as a guide only. If other points are clearly more tender, or are strongly indicated by a point locator, they should be considered as preferable alternatives.

In some formulae, the points suggested are close together, and may be detected as a single point, which should be used.

Dermal

Like the press needles, the dermal needles are intended to remain in the skin. They are usually made of silver and are about $\frac{1}{2}$ inch long, and straight. Another type, made of stainless steel, resembles a flattened press needle with a longer shank. Both types of dermal needle are inserted obliquely through the skin, so as not to completely penetrate the skin. They may be left in position for not longer than one week, protected by adhesive plaster, as shown in Figure 30.

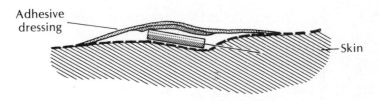

Figure 30
Implanted dermal needle

The skin surface should be cleaned thoroughly before a sterile dermal needle is implanted. The patient should be told to remove the dressing and the needle at the slightest sign of soreness or infection. The dermal needle often leaves a small lump on the skin. This normally disappears within a day.

Dermal needles may be inserted in acupuncture points, or in painful spots which may not be acupuncture points. In a painful area, up to six needles may be implanted. Edemas, skin eruptions and rashes must be strictly avoided.

A dermal needle may be left in a particularly important point which has been used in the regular treatment, for example SP 6 or ST 36. This is not necessarily the most effective use of this type of needle. An alternative is to use the *Xi*-cleft points[1] which are:

HT 6	PC 4	LU 6
SI 6	TH 7	CO 7
BL 63	GB 36	ST 34
KI 5	LI 6	SP 8

[1] Dr K. Yamawaki, *Dermal Needle Therapy*, 1975.

In addition, four of the eight extra meridians have *Xi*-cleft points, which are recommended for acute conditions only:

Yinchaiomo	KI 8	For female organic and fluid problems.
Yinweimo	KI 9	For kidney, *Yuan chi* deficient, and cold diseases.
Yangchaiomo	BL 59	For rheumatic conditions, especially in males.
Yangweimo	GB 35	For migraine, headache, genital and hot diseases.

Other special dermal needle points are:

LU 1	(Needle in direction of energy flow) to stimulate lungs for chronic skin, lung and throat conditions.
PC 1	(Needle in direction of energy flow) for chronic chest, heart, stomach and arm conditions, in males only.
VC 17	(Needle upwards) for chronic breathing conditions, asthma, bronchitis etc.
VC 12	(Needle downwards) for stomach ulcers.
LI 13	(Needle upwards) for chronic dysentry and diarrhoea.
GB 25	(Needle downwards) to sedate kidney.
VC 14	(Needle upwards) for chronic heart conditions, palpitations, etc.

SYMPTOMATIC TREATMENTS

Anal Fissure

Main points	GV 1, GV 11, BL 54, CO 4, LI 9.
Ear points	*Shenmen*, lower rectum, large intestine, spleen.
Needleless	GV 20, VC 6, VC 8, VC 12.
Press needle	*Shenmen*, lower rectum.
Dermal	CO 7.

Anal Prolapse

Main points	GV 1, GV 20, BL 57, ST 36, SP 6.
Additionals	VC 6, VC 8.
Ear points	*Shenmen*, lower rectum, large intestine, spleen.
Needleless	GV 20, VC 6, VC 8, VC 12, ST 36, ST 37, ST 38.
Press needle	*Shenmen*, lower rectum.
Dermal	CO 7.

Anaemia

Main points	VC 12, CO 11, ST 36, PC 6, LU 7.
Additionals	BL 18, BL 19, BL 39, GV 13.
Ear points	Spleen, endocrine, sympathy.
Needleless	SP 4, SP 8, CO 10, CO 11, VC 12, ST 36, LU 7, LU 9, BL 20.
Press needle	Sympathy, spleen.
Dermal	ST 34.

Use two points with strong stimulation.

Angina Pectoris

Main points	PC 6 (through to TH 5), ST 36.
Additionals	PC 5, BL 17, LI 13, VC 17.
	For chronic cases CO 2, CO 4, PC 2, LU 10 (all stimulate), plus CO 11 (sedate).
Ear points	Heart, sympathy, thorax.
Needleless	PC 3, PC 4, PC 6, PC 7, LU 9, KI 3, BL 15, BL 66, VC 14.
Press needle	Sympathy, thorax.
Dermal	PC 4.
Moxa	During attack, moxa VC 17. See also Chapter Seven.

Amenorrhoea

Main points	VC 3, VC 4, SP 6, SP 10, ST 36.
Additionals	KI 8, CO 4, BL 18, VC 6.
Ear Points	Adrenal, *Shenmen*, kidney, endocrine, sympathy.
Needleless	ST 29, SP 9, KI 11.
Press needle	Adrenal, kidney.
Dermal	KI 8.
Moxa	See Chapter Seven.

Ankle, sprained

Main points	BL 60, KI 3, ST 41, GB 39, LI 3.
Ear points	Ankle, liver, subcortex.
Needleless	ST 41, ST 42, GB 39.
Press needle	Subcortex, ankle.
Dermal	BL 59.
Moxa	See Chapter Seven.

Appendicitis

Main points	*Lanwei*, ST 36, CO 11, ST 44, ST 25.
Ear points	Appendix (back of auricle).
	Appendix (*cymba conchai*).
	Appendix 1, sympathy, stomach.
Needleless	ST 36, CO 11, ST 43, ST 44, TH 5, TH 6, BL 54.
Press needle	Sympathy, appendix (rear auricle).
Dermal	None.

Arm Pains
Main points	*Chienneilung*, CO 4, CO 11, CO 15, SI 10, TH 14.
Additionals	*Chingpi*, CO 14, CO 12, SI 11, HT 1.
Ear points	Elbow, shoulder, wrist, kidney, subcortex.
Needleless	According to location of pain.
Press needle	Subcortex, shoulder.
Dermal	SI 6.

Arthritis – Rheumatoid
Main points	BL 11, BL 58, CO 4, CO 11, CO 15, TH 5.
Ear points	Kidney, *Pingchuan*, internal secretion, adrenal, *Shenmen*, Subcortex.
Needleless	GB 38.
Press needle	Internal secretion, kidney.
Dermal	None.

Arthritis – Osteo-Arthritis
Main points	BL 23, SP 5, TH 4, TH 15, KI 6.
Ear points	Kidney, internal secretion, *Shenmen* subcortex, adrenal.
Needleless	GB 38.
Press needle	Adrenal, kidney.
Dermal	None.

Arthritis: Additional local treatments
Neck and Spine
Main points	*Paiao*, *Chichingchinpang*, TH 3, GV 20.
Ear points	Neck, clavicle.
Needleless	TH 12, TH 14, GB 19, TH 16, GV 13, CO 18.

Shoulder
Main points	CO 15, TH 14, HT 1, SI 9.
Ear points	Shoulder, shoulder joint, clavicle.
Needleless	ST 19, CO 14, TH 11, SI 9.
Moxa	See Chapter Seven.

Elbow
Main points	GB 9, LU 5, CO 11, TH 5.
Ear points	Elbow.
Needleless	CO 11, PC 6, TH 3.

Wrist
Main points	TH 4, TH 5, TH 6, CO 4, LU 5.
Ear points	Wrist.
Needleless	LU 9.

Fingers
Main points	*Shangpahsieh*, *Szufeng*, LU 7, TH 4.
Ear points	Wrist, fingers.
Needleless	TH 3, TH 4, PC 8.

Lumbo-sacral
Main points   *Shichichuihsia*, GV 3.
Ear points   Lumbo-sacral.
Needleless   GB 27, GB 39, SP 4, SP 8, GV 3, GV 4.
Moxa   See Chapter Seven.

Sacro-iliac
Main points   BL 25, BL 27.
Ear points   Lumbo-sacral, buttock.
Needleless   BL 26, BL 27, BL 29, BL 30, BL 31, BL 32, BL 33, BL 34, BL 48.
Moxa   See Chapter Seven.

Hip
Main points   BL 37, BL 54, GB 30, GB 34, KI 8, GV 1.
Ear points   Buttock, hip, *ku-kuan*.

Knee
Main points   *Hsiyen* (both sides), *Heting*, ST 34, GB 34, BL 54, SP 6, SP 10, ST 35, ST 36.
Ear points   Knee.
Needleless   *Weishing, Hsiwai, Hsiyen, Hsihsia*, BL 53, BL 54.

Ankle
Main points   GB 39, GB 40, LI 3, LI 4, ST 41, KI 3, BL 60, BL 62.
Ear points   Ankle.
Needleless   ST 41, ST 42.
Moxa   See Chapter Seven.

Foot and Toes
Main points   *Pafeng.*
Ear points   Toes.
Needleless   *Pafeng*, ST 41, ST 42.
Press needle   *Pingchuan*, toes.
Dermal   For acute cases, males only, BL 59.

Anxiety Neurosis and Nervous Tension
Main points   HT 7, SP 6, PC 6, *Taiyang, Paihui.*
Ear points   Subcortex, *Shenmen*, heart, kidney.
Needleless   GV 12, GB 20, VC 6, VC 7, HT 3, HT 7, PC 6.
Press needle   *Shenmen.*
Dermal   None.

Asthma (see also Bronchial Asthma)

Main points	BL 13, BL 17, VC 17, LU 7, Chienchuan, Chuanhsi.
	Acute attacks males – VC 22, ST 12; females – VC 22, BL 12, GB 21.
Additionals	GV 14, BL 60, ST 44, VC 4, plus moxa VC 6.
Ear points	Shenmen, lung, adrenal, asthma, sympathy.
Needleless	LU 5, LU 8, ST 10, CO 20, ST 12, ST 19, ST 21, VC 17.
Press needle	Adrenal, asthma.

Back Pain

Main points	Chiachi points, SI 3, BL 51.
Ear points	Cervical vertebra, lumbar vertebra, kidney, Shenmen.
Needleless	LU 1, LU 5, LU 8, CO 8, ST 10, ST 19, SP 21, KI 3.
Press needles	Subcortex, plus local point.
Implant	BL 59.

Bronchial Asthma

Main points	VC 17, VC 22, BL 13, BL 17.
Additionals	ST 40, GB 20, VC 12, PC 3, CO 4, KI 8, LU 9.
Ear points	Pingchuan, endocrine, Shenmen, lung.
Needleless	LU 1, LU 5, LU 8, CO 8, ST 10, ST 19, SP 21, KI 3.
Press needles	Pingchuan, lung.
Dermal	LU 1.

Bronchitis (and Infections of the Upper Respiratory Tract)

Chronic

Main points	BL 13, Chuanhsi, VC 22, PC 6, ST 40, KI 6, LU 1, LU 7.
Additionals	Chiachi points from C.6 to Th.4, GV 14.
Ear points	Adrenal, Shenmen, parotid.
Needleless	LU 1, ST 10, ST 13, BL 13, KI 22, KI 25, KI 26.
Press needles	Shenmen.
Dermal	LU 1.
Moxa	See Chapter Seven.

Acute

Main points	LU 5, TH 3, ST 40, CO 4, LU 7, VC 17, VC 20.
Additionals	Chiachi points from C.6 to Th.4, GV 14, cough point (hand).
Ear points	Lung, adrenal, Ku-Kuan, parotid.
Needleless	ST 10, ST 13, KI 25, KI 26, KI 27, PC 3, TH 10.
Press needles	Pingchuan, lung.
Dermal	LU 1.

Common Cold

Main points	GB 20, BL 12, TH 5, CO 4, GV 20.
With headache	Add *Taiyang, Intang.*
With fever	Add CO 11, GV 14, ST 36.
With high fever	Add GV 13, ST 43.
With stuffy nose	Add CO 20, BL 7, GV 19.
With sore throat	Add LU 11 (prick to bleeding).
Ear points	*Shenmen*, sympathy, lung, *Pinchuan.*
Needleless	BL 12, GB 20, GV 13, GV 20, CO 11, ST 36.
Press needles	Adrenal.
Dermal	GB 35.
Moxa	See Chapter Seven.

Conjunctivitis

Main points	Taiyang (prick till bleeding).
	BL 1, CO 4, GB 14, GB 20, LU 11.
Additionals	GV 1, GB 24, GB 34, CO 2, KI 18, KI 6.
Ear points	Lung, liver, eye 1, eye 2.
Needleless	ST 36, SI 19, BL 18, TH 20, TH 22, GB 14.
Press needles	Liver, eye 1, eye 2.
Dermal	None.
Moxa	See Chapter Seven.

Constipation

Main points	TH 6, ST 25, VC 6, BL 21, ST 40.
Additionals	GV 1, GB 24, GB 34, CO 2, KI 6, KI 18.
Ear points	Stomach, abdomen, sympathy, large intestine, small intestine.
Needleless	*Chronic* KI 16, GB 24.
	Acute ST 22, ST 36, GB 34, SP 5, SP 15, KI 8, KI 19, LI 1, LI 2.
Press needles	Endocrine, abdomen.
Dermal	KI 9.
Moxa	See Chapter Seven.

Cough

Main points	LU 5, LU 7, LU 9, *Chuanhsi, Chienchuan*, BL 13.
Additionals	KI 3, BL 60, CO 4.
Ear points	*Shenmen*, adrenal, lung, larynx, *Pingchuan.*
Needleless	LU 6, CO 18, ST 9, ST 11, ST 17, ST 18, ST 19, ST 20, KI 1, KI 3, GB 41, ST 43.
Press needles	*Pingchuan*, cough (rear of auricle).
Dermal	LU 6.
Moxa	See Chapter Seven.

Deafness

Main points	TH 3, TH 17, GV 23, SI 19.
Ear points	Kidney, *Pingchuan*, internal ear, external ear.
Needleless	GB 20, TH 17, SI 19.
Press needle	Internal ear.
Dermal	None.

Depression (Reactive, i.e., with Reasonable Cause)

Main points	HT 3, HT 9, PC 6, SP 6, VC 15, GV 19, LU 5.
Ear points	Heart, brain, kidney, *Shenmen, Pingchuan,* stomach, subcortex, uterus.
Needleless	TH 10, ST 41, BL 10.
Press needle	*Shenmen.*
Dermal	None.

Diarrhoea

Main points	VC 12, ST 36, CO 2, CO 4, CO 11.
Additionals	*Acute* ST 25, ST 26, ST $26\frac{1}{2}$ (needle) ST $25\frac{1}{2}$, ST 27 (moxa).
	Temperature GV 14, CO 11.
	Stomach pain LI 3, TH 8.
	'Runs' VC 13, ST 25, ST 26.
Ear points	Large intestine, *Shenmen,* liver, gall bladder, subcortex.
Needleless	ST 20, GV 3.
Press needles	*Shenmen,* gall bladder.
Implant	LI 13.

Dysmenorrhoea

Main points	SP 6, LI 3, VC 4, VC 6, ST 36, KI 8, BL 31.
Ear points	Sympathy, internal secretion, *Shenmen,* subcortex.
Needleless	VC 4, ST 27.
Press needles	Endocrine plus uterus (during or after period), or Ovary (during period).
Dermal	KI 8.

Eczema

Main points	GV 14, SP 6, CO 11.
Ear points	*Shenmen,* lung, liver, subcortex.
Needleless	BL 10, CO 15, BL 13, VF 12, CO 11, KI 9.
Press needles	*Shenmen,* local points.
Dermal	LI 1.

Edema

Main points	SP 9, GV 26, KI 7.
Ear points	*Shenmen,* sympathy, adrenal, kidney, bladder.
Needleless	ST 40, SP 9, KI 8, LI 5, LI 9.
Press needles	Adrenal, bladder.
Dermal	KI 9.

Elbow Pains

Main points	CO 11, CO 12, TH 10, LU 3, PC 6.
Ear points	Subcortex, kidney, elbow.
Needleless	SI 4, CO 11.
Press needles	Elbow, subcortex.
Dermal	CO 7.

Enteritis

Main points	ST 25, ST 27, ST 36, VC 4, VC 6, *Moxa* VC 4 and VC 6.
Additionals	*Nausea* PC 6.
	Pain ST 34.
	Fever GV 4, CO 4, CO 11, BL 22, GV 13.
	Vomiting LI 3, LI 14.
	Diarrhoea SP 4, SP 6.
Ear points	Apex of auricle, sympathy, large intestine, small intestine, gastro-intestinal.
Needleless	ST 22, ST 23, ST 24, ST 38.
Press needles	Apex of auricle, large intestine.
Dermal	LI 13.
Moxa	See Chapter Seven.

Eye Problems

Main points	*Taiyang,* ST 1, ST 2, ST 36, BL 1, BL 2, BL 18, GB 1, TH 23, *Yiming, Yuyau, Chiuhou.*
Ear points	Liver, eye 1, eye 2.
Needleless	ST 36, SI 19, BL 18, TH 20, GB 14.
Dermal	None.
Moxa	See Chapter Seven.

Fever

Main points	GV 13, GV 14, CO 11, TH 5.
Ear points	*Shenmen,* adrenal, occiput, subcortex.
Needleless	CO 11, CO 4, TH 5, GV 14.
Press needles	*Shenmen.*
Dermal	GB 35.

Gall Stones

Main points	BL 19, VC 12, PC 6, ST 36.
Ear points	Sympathy, *Shenmen,* gall bladder, duodenum, liver, subcortex.
Needleless	None.
Press needles	*Shenmen,* gall bladder.
Dermal	GB 36.

Gastritis

Main points	TH 6, ST 36, VC 12, BL 21, *Chiachi* points from Th.8 to Th.12.
Ear points	Stomach, subcortex.
Needleless	ST 34, VC 12, BL 45, LI 13, VC 10, ST 21, ST 19.
Press needles	Stomach, subcortex.
Dermal	LI 13.
Moxa	See Chapter Seven.

Goitre
Main points	CO 4, ST 9, PC 6, SP 6, TH 13, *Chiyang* (two needles each side of thyroid mass).
Ear points	Adrenal, subcortex, endocrine, *Shenmen*.
Needleless	GB 20, BL 10, GV 12, CO 18, LU 5, VC 12, ST 9.
Press needles	Adrenal.
Dermal	None.

Gout
Main points	BL 19, BL 23, TH 5, VC 4, SP 6.
Ear points	*Shenmen*, adrenal, *Pinchuan*, internal secretion, apex of auricle, kidney, toes.
Needleless	None.
Press needles	Internal secretion, toes.
Dermal	None.

Haemorrhoids
Main points	GV 1, BL 50, SP 5, SP 6, BL 57, LI 13.
Ear points	*Shenmen*, large intestine, lower rectum.
Needleless	SP 5, GV 1, GV 2, GV 3, GV 4, GV 20, LU 6, BL 32.
Press needle	*Shenmen*, lower rectum.
Dermal	GB 35.
Moxa	See Chapter Seven.

Headaches
Main points	GB 20, GV 20, LI 3, BL 65, *Yuyao*.
Additionals	*Back of head* BL 10, SI 3, GV 14.
	Temporal GB 8, TH 3, GB 41, *Taiyang*.
	Forehead ST 41, CO 4, GB 14, *Yintang*.
Ear points	Subcortex, forehead, back of head, headache 1, 2 and 3 (back of auricle).
Needleless	GV 11, GV 16, GV 18, CO 4, CO 5, CO 14, ST 36, HT 2.
Press needles	Subcortex, local point.
Dermal	None.

Hay Fever
Main points	GV 19, GV 23, GV 25, CO 20, *Yintang*, CO 4, LU 7.
Ear points	Adrenal, internal secretion, subcortex.
Needleless	SP 4, CO 4, KI 15.
Press needles	Adrenal.
Dermal	CO 7.

Heartburn
Main points	VC 10, ST 12, HT 9, LI 9, LI 13.
Ear points	Stomach, duodenum, sympathy.
Needleless	ST 11, ST 21, ST 36, ST 37, SP 16, VC 4.
Press needles	Sympathy, stomach.
Dermal	ST 34 or LI 13.
Moxa	See Chapter Seven.

Heartstroke
Main points	CO 11, GV 14, GV 26, KI 1, BL 54, *Shixuan*.
Ear point	*Shenmen*.
Needleless	CO 11, KI 3.
Press needle	*Shenmen*.
Dermal	None.

Hemiplegia
Main points	CO 4, CO 11, CO 15, TH 5, GB 30, GB 31, GB 34, GB 39.
Ear points	Adrenal, *Shenmen*, sympathy.
Needleless	LI 4.
Press needle	*Shenmen*.
Dermal	None.

Hernia
Main points	ST 30, LI 3.
Ear points	Subcortex, liver, spleen, testes or ovary.
Needleless	None.
Press needle	Subcortex, testes or ovary.
Dermal	GB 35.

Hives (Urticaria)
Main points	LI 2, LI 13, LI 14, SP 6, SP 10, ST 36.
Ear points	Liver, urticaria, *Shenmen*, subcortex, adrenal.
Needleless	BL 12, BL 17, BL 20, CO 15, CO 11, CO 10.
Press needle	Urticaria, liver.
Dermal	LI 6.

Impotence
Main points	VC 2, VC 3, VC 4, VC 6, GV 4, BL 23, LI 5, LI 8.
Ear points	Endocrine, *Shenmen*, adrenal, liver, kidney.
Needleless	None.
Press needles	Adrenal, liver.
Dermal	GB 35.

Hypertension
Main points	GV 20, GB 20, CO 11, ST 36, *Taiyang*, *Yintang*, TH 17.
Ear points	Depressing groove, *Shenmen*, subcortex, high blood pressure, sympathy.
Needleless	BL 47, LI 14, CO 11, CO 4, ST 27, ST 36, VC 12.
Press needles	Depressing groove, subcortex.
Dermal	None.

Indigestion

Main points	VC 6, VC 12, BL 20, BL 23, SP 6.
Additionals	*'Nervous stomach'* VC 11, ST 25, ST 36, BL 54, Moxa GV 3.
	Acidity Gall bladder points.
	Vomiting PC 6, VC 22.
Ear points	Stomach, internal secretion, gall bladder, large intestine, small intestine.
Needleless	ST 11, ST 21, ST 36, ST 37, SP 3, SP 16, LI 13, VC 4, VC 5.
Press needles	Internal secretion, stomach.
Dermal	ST 34.
Moxa	See Chapter Seven.

Influenza

Main points	CO 4, GV 13, GV 20, GV 14, GB 20.
Additionals	*Stuffy nose* CO 20.
	Sweating KI 7.
	Fever CO 11.
	Cough LU 7, BL 12.
	Sore throat Bleed LU 11.
Ear points	Adrenal, subcortex, *Shenmen, Pingchuan*, lung.
Needleless	ST 36, CO 4, GB 20, GV 16.
Press needles	*Shenmen*, lung.
Dermal	LU 1.
Moxa	See Chapter Seven.

Insomnia

Main points	*Yiming*, BL 15, HT 7, PC 6, SP 6.
Ear points	Subcortex, *Shenmen, Pingchuan*, sympathy, heart, kidney.
Needleless	Liver or spleen points.
Press needles	*Shenmen*, heart.
Dermal	None.

Laryngitis

Main points	VC 22, GB 20, CO 4, CO 20, BL 12, ST 40, GV 14, SI 1, *Taiyang, Chiachi* points from Th.1 to Th.3.
Ear points	*Shenmen*, internal secretion, heart, pharynx, larynx.
Needleless	CO 2, ST 10, ST 11, TH 9, TH 10, TH 16, GB 20, KI 3, LU 5.
Press needles	*Shenmen*, pharynx and larynx.
Dermal	LU 1.

Leg Pains

Main points	GB 29, GB 31, LI 11, GB 41.
Ear points	Adrenal, gall bladder, knee, ankle, liver.
Needleless	ST 36, ST 42, ST 45, SP 1, SP 5, SP 6.
Press needles	Adrenal, local points.
Dermal	GB 36.

Lumbago

Main points	*Huatuojiaji, moxa* BL 23, BL 25, BL 50, BL 60, GV 26, GV 4, GB 30, SI 3, LI 11.
Ear points	*Shenmen*, internal secretion, kidney, subcortex, lower back (back of auricle), lumbago (back of auricle).
Needleless	BL 54, BL 23, KI 7.
Press needles	Internal secretion, lumbago.
Dermal	BL 59.
Moxa	For other moxa treatment, see Chapter Seven.

Mastitis

Main points	ST 18, LI 3.
Ear points	Chest, stomach, kidney, sympathy.
Needleless	ST 18.
Press needle	Chest sympathy.
Dermal	None.

Menopausal syndromes

Main points	BL 32, BL 39, VC 6, SP 6.
Ear points	Sympathy, *Shenmen*, internal secretion, uterus.
Needleless	BL 10, BL 12, BL 15, VC 4, VC 6, VC 12.
Press needle	Sympathy, uterus.
Dermal	KI 8.

Menstrual Irregularity

Main points	VC 2, VC 3, VC 4, VC 6, BL 23, SP 9, SP 10, ST 36.
Ear points	Subcortex, endocrine, sympathy, uterus, ovary.
Needleless	BL 10, SP 10, KI 5, KI 6, KI 13, LI 9, KI 14, GB 26, SP 6.
Press needle	Endocrine, ovary.
Dermal	KI 8.

Migraine

Main points	CO 4, LU 7, GV 20, GB 20, *Taiyang, Yuyuo*.
Ear points	*Pingchuan*, subcortex, apex of auricle, *Shenmen*, liver.
Needleless	ST 36, GB 20, LI 3, *Taiyang, Yeeming*.
Press needles	*Shenmen*, liver.
Dermal	GB 36.

Morning Sickness

Main points	PC 6, ST 36.
Ear points	*Shenmen*, sympathy, endocrine, stomach, duodenum.
Needleless	PC 6, VC 11, ST 25, *In-tang*.
Press needles	Endocrine, stomach.
Dermal	ST 34.

Neck (Stiff or Sprained)

Main points	GB 20, GB 39, SI 6, *Ahshi* points.
Ear points	Kidney, neck, small intestine.
Needleless	CO 18, ST 11, SI 16.
Press needles	Neck.
Dermal	None.

Nervous Tension (see also Anxiety and Depression)

Main points	GB 39, ST 36, VC 15, GV 19, LI 13.
Ear points	*Shenmen*, sympathy, lung, forehead, kidney, stomach.
Needleless	GV 12, VC 6, HT 3, HT 7, LI 3, CO 4.
Press needles	*Shenmen*.
Dermal	GB 35.

Neurosis

Main points	GV 15, BL 13, BL 23, KI 3.
Ear points	Subcortex, occiput, kidney, *Shenmen*.
Needleless	SP 1, SI 1, ST 23, HT 3.
Press needles	*Shenmen*.
Dermal	None.

Neurodermatitis

Main points	CO 4, CO 11, SP 6, SP 10.
Ear points	*Shenmen*, adrenal, subcortex, lung, liver.
Needleless	None.
Press needles	*Shenmen*, lung.
Dermal	None.

Paraplegia

Main points	*Chiachi* points BL 32, BL 49, LI 11, BL 54, *Linghou*, ST 36, SP 6.
Ear points	*Shenmen*, adrenal, subcortex, brain.
Needleless	ST 34, ST 36, ST 38, SI 9, KI 7, GB 43.
Press needles	*Shenmen*, brain.
Dermal	None.

Pneumonia

Main points	BL 12, BL 13.
Ear points	*Shenmen*, sympathy, lung, *Pingchuan*.
Needleless	ST 13, SP 18, SP 21.
Press needles	*Shenmen*, lung.
Dermal	LU 1.
Moxa	See Chapter Seven.

Pleurisy

Main points	BL 12, BL 13.
Ear points	*Shenmen*, sympathy, adrenal, lung, chest.
Needleless	None.
Press needles	*Shenmen*, lung.
Dermal	LU 1.

Prolapse

Main points	SP 6, VC 3, VC 4, needle and moxa.
Ear points	Subcortex, uterus, *Shenmen*, external genitals.
Needleless	KI 1.
Press needles	Subcortex, uterus.
Dermal	KI 8.

Rhinitis

Main points	BL 7, *Yintang*, ST 2, CO 4, CO 19, CO 20.
Ear points	Internal nose, adrenal, internal secretion.
Needleless	CO 19, CO 20, ST 3, CO 4, BL 10.
Press needles	*Shenmen*, internal nose.
Dermal	CO 7.

Sinusitis

Main points	CO 20, BL 2, ST 2, BL 7, *Taiyang*, GB 20.
Ear points	Adrenal, lung, *Shenmen*, subcortex.
Needleless	CO 4, CO 20, *Taiyang*.
Press needles	*Shenmen*, internal nose.
Dermal	GB 35.

Sciatica

Main points	*Chiachi* points, lumbar 4 and 5, GB 30, GB 34, *Linghoui*, plus bladder points.
Ear points	*Shenmen, Ischium*, buttock, *Pingchuan*, lumbar vert., sacral vert.
Needleless	BL 54, BL 60, GV 4 (same side as pain).
Press needles	*Shenmen*, sacral vertebra.
Dermal	BL 59.

Shock

Main points	GV 26, *Shihhsuan*, KI 1, ST 36, PC 6, VC 6.
Ear points	*Shenmen*, adrenal, heart, lung.
Needleless	GV 26, KI 1.
Press needles	Adrenal, lung.
Dermal	None.

Shoulder Pain

Main points	Local SI, CO and TH points, GB 34, TH 6, *Yanglingchuan, Chienneilung.*
Ear points	Subcortex, shoulder, shoulder joint, kidney.
Needleless	Local points.
Press needles	Subcortex, shoulder.
Dermal	Local painful places.
Moxa	See Chapter Seven.

Stomach Pain

Main points	VC 8 (moxa), PC 6, SP 4, VC 12, ST 25, TH 8, LI 3.
Additionals	'Hot' conditions DT 43, ST 45.
	'Cold' conditions VC 4, VC 14 (moxa), BL 20, ST 36, VC 6.
	Overeating VC 11, VC 21, ST 36, ST 44.
Ear points	Abdomen, stomach, sympathy.
Needleless	ST 34, ST 21, ST 36, SP 2, SP 12, SP 16, KI 16.
Press needles	Sympathy, stomach.
Dermal	VC 12 (downwards).
Moxa	See Chapter Seven.

Stroke

Main points	GV 26, CO 4, SP 6, VC 4, VC 6, VC 8.
Ear points	Brain, *Pingchuan*, subcortex, kidney, adrenal.
Needleless	None.
Press needles	Adrenal, brain.
Dermal	None.

Tinnitis

Main points	TH 17, TH 21, SI 19, SI 3, CO 4, GB 20, TH 5, *Yiming.*
Ear points	Kidney, *Pingchuan*, internal ear.
Needleless	CO 1, CO 4, CO 5, CO 6, plus local points.
Press needles	*Pingchuan*, internal ear.
Dermal	None.

Toothache

Main points	ST 6, ST 7, ST 44, VC 24, CO 4, *Pahsieh, Shangpahsieh.*
Ear points	Tooth anaesthesia points 1 and 2, large intestine, adrenal.
Needleless	CO 4.
Press needles	Tooth anaesthesia points 1 and 2.
Dermal	None.
Moxa	See Chapter Seven.

Tonsillitis

Main points	SI 17, CO 4, LU 11, ST 44, VC 17.
Ear points	Tonsils 1, 2 and 4, Helix 1 and 6, pharynx-larynx, adrenal.
Needleless	CO 2, CO 17, ST 10, ST 11, TH 9, TH 10, GB 20.
Press needles	Adrenal, pharynx-larynx.
Dermal	None.

Trigeminal Neuralgia

Main points	*Taiyang, Chiachenchiang,* ST 2, ST 4, ST 7, CO 4, ST 44, LI 3, ST 36.
Ear points	Forehead, Maxilla, Mandibula, *Shenmen*, sympathy, *Hsia-he*.
Needleless	ST 3, *Taiyang*, ST 5, CO 4, *Yeeming*.
Press needles	*Shenmen*.
Dermal	None.

Ulcers (Duodenal)

Main points	VC 15, ST 12, ST 36, CO 4, VC 4, VC 12, GV 19.
Ear points	Duodenum, stomach, sympathy, *Shenmen*, subcortex, ulcer (rear of auricle).
Needleless	VC 12, PC 6, ST 36.
Press needles	Sympathy, ulcer.
Dermal	VC 12 (downwards).

Ulcers (Gastric)

Main points	CO 4, VC 12, VC 15, ST 12, ST 25, ST 36.
Ear points	Ulcer (back of auricle), stomach, sympathy, *Shenmen*, subcortex.
Needleless	VC 12, PC 6, ST 36.
Press needles	Sympathy, stomach.
Dermal	VC 12 (downwards).

Urinary Problems

Main points	VC 3, VC 4, VC 6, BL 31, BL 32, SP 6, LI 8, CO 11.
Ear points	*Sanjaio*, sympathy, kidney, bladder, urethra.
Needleless	BL 31, BL 32, SP 6.
Press needles	Sympathy, *Sanjaio*.
Dermal	KI 9.
Moxa	See Chapter Seven.

Uterine Problems

Main points   CO 4, SP 6, CO 11, VC 16, ST 25.
Ear points   Sympathy, endocrine, kidney, uterus, ovary.
Needleless   ST 25, ST 28, ST 30, KI 13, GB 28, GB 29, plus moxa
                 VC 4.
Press needles Endocrine, uterus.
Dermal   KI 8.

7

Special Moxibustion Points

Many western acupuncturists tend to regard the use of moxa as a 'second-best' treatment, and use it only when the use of needles is impractical. Others use moxa only for certain well-defined 'cold' diseases.

In fact, moxibustion is sometimes more effective than needles. This is so when the treatment is applied to normal acupuncture points. But moxa treatments need not be confined to acupuncture points. In this chapter, a series of treatments are described which use points not shown on charts, and which are not used for needle acupuncture. The points which are shown on *Newest Illustrations of Acupuncture Points* as 'Strange' or 'New' points are named accordingly.

Modern practice is replacing the traditional method of moxibustion by burning small piles of moxa on the skin, with the use of the more convenient moxa tube. This is usually a paper roll of compressed moxa about the size of a cigar. New methods of applying heat to localized points on the skin are also being introduced. These seem to be reasonably effective, so it may be no more than prejudice on the part of the authors that they still prefer moxa tubes.

In each case, an indication is given as to the duration of the treatment. This is necessarily variable. A heavy person with a chronic condition will need longer treatments than a very lightweight person with an acute condition. The time given is for the total treatment of all the points suggested. When using other forms of heating appliance, the manufacturers' instructions should be followed.

It is the practice of the authors to encourage the patient to treat himself between visits. The patient is provided with a supply of moxa rolls and explicit written instructions. The latter is essential as a patient cannot be expected to remember treatment details.

Internal Organic Diseases of the Yin Organs
The treatment of any disease in which the *Yin* energy of the

organs is weak, can be helped by the daily application of moxibustion to a point on the sternum midway between VC 15 and VC 16. Some caution is required as this point has a strong stimulant effect on the heart. One to two minutes is sufficient.

General Weakness

When a condition of weakness calls for the stimulation of *Yang* energy, use moxa on the crease between the sacrum and the ilium which is formed when the patient is standing. This is the channel for a strong flow of *Yang* energy which can be strengthened by moxa. Treatment may be from 5 to 10 minutes.

Heart Pains

There is a branch from the Main colon meridian. This leaves the Main meridian 2 *tsun* above the wrist flexure and terminates at the end of the middle finger. The point *Chungchuan* on this branch, is at the wrist flexure, between TH 4 and CO 5. For heart pains, and any other hot symptoms of the internal organs, moxa for 4 to 6 minutes.

Abdominal Pains (see Figure 31)

The moxa treatment for abdominal pains is applied at the lumbar region, and in the area of the big toe.

Lumbar region
GV 4, BL 25, BL 27 (needle).
Tip of the process of the 3rd lumbar vertebra may be moxa'ed as long as necessary.

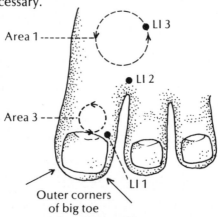

Area 1 ---- •LI 3

•LI 2

Area 3 --

LI 1

Outer corners
of big toe

Figure 31
Big toe points for moxa treatment of abdominal pains

Big toe area
    (1) Start from LI 3 and move the moxa tube in a circle over the area of the first metatarsal.
    (2) LI 1, LI 2.
    (3) Area at the root of the big toe nail.
    (4) The outer corners of the big toe nail.

Treat bilaterally for a total of 10 to 12 minutes, expending most time on areas (1) and (4).

Intestinal Troubles
Moxa the tip of the elbow, and CO 11, for 6 to 8 minutes. For acute conditions, also moxa along the stomach meridians from ST 25 to ST 27 for 6 to 8 minutes.

Coughs and Gastralgia
This treatment is more suitable for males. Use moxa for 4 to 6 minutes to heat a circular area, $1\frac{1}{2}$ inches diameter, directly below the aureola of each nipple.

Indigestion
For acute indigestion, moxa the tips of the fingers and thumb of one hand. Treat the left hand for men, right hand for women. Continue until the pain subsides, which may take 15 minutes or longer. Pricking the tips usually accelerates the cure.

Loss of Appetitie
The special moxibustion points are, firstly, bilateral and $\frac{1}{2}$ *tsun* lateral to SP 15. This is level with the umbilicus. The second point is on the left side of the body only, and $\frac{1}{2}$ *tsun* lateral to VC 12. To stimulate appetite, moxa the above points for 6 minutes, then moxa BL 21 for 12 minutes.
If needling may also be employed, there is a special point on the left side of the body only, on the axilla. It is anterior to HT 1 and immediately posterior to the pectoral muscle. Tonification of this point at a depth of .8 to 1 inch has a powerful stimulating effect on the appetite.

Constipation
Treat with moxa for 4 to 6 minutes, bilaterally, exactly 1 *tsun* each side of the umbilicus. Then, with the patient's mouth open, apply the moxa roll once only at each corner of the mouth.

Diarrhoea
Treat for 3 to 5 minutes with moxa at point *Yaochi*, which is on the medial line of the sacrum, at a level midway between the second and third foramen.

Haemorrhoids
Treat four points between the anus and GV 3. These are:

(1) *Yaochi*, midway between the levels of the second and third foramen. Treat for 5 minutes.
(2) A point midway between GV 1 and GV 2. Treat for 10 minutes.
(3) GV 1. Treat for 1 minute.
(4) The posterior edge of the anus. Treat for 10 minutes.

Bronchitis, Pneumonia and All Chest Conditions
Treat with moxa for 15 to 20 minutes in the region of the 4th thoracic vertebra. Pass the tip of the moxa roll from BL 13 on one side to BL 13 on the other, passing over the process of the 4th thoracic vertebra, and GV 12.

Fluid Retention
These problems, which commonly resist other forms of treatment, may respond to moxa treatment of the second toe, at the centre of the first phalanx. 8 to 10 minutes, as frequently as possible.

When the retention of fluid is due to diabetes, a special point on the edge of the plantar skin of the foot, directly below the internal malleolus, should be moxa'ed daily for 4 to 6 minutes.

Bladder Problems
Treat with the tip of the 3rd lumbar vertebra, and BL 28. Moxa from 5 to 15 minutes.

Nephritis (Inflamation of the Kidney)
Moxa for 2 to 5 minutes, bilaterally, at a point anterior to SP 10 at the outer edge of the sartoris muscle.

Female Genital Problems
There are two pairs of adjacent bilateral points which are applicable to all such problems:

(1) SP 6 and *Chengming*, which is 1 *tsun* posterior to SP 6.
(2) The centre of the phalanx of the big toe, and the area at the root of the nail of the big toe (Area 3 on Fig. 31).

Moxa each pair of points 6 to 8 minutes.

Dysmenorrhoea
Treat by slowly moving the tip of the moxa roll round the internal malleolus at a distance of $\frac{1}{2}$ to 1 *tsun* from the tip of the malleolus. Total treatment time 8 to 10 minutes. Additional treatment is moxibustion along the webs of the toes from LI 2 to GB 43. Total treatment time 4 to 6 minutes.

Excessive Menstruation
Moxa two points on each foot:

(1) The dorsal surface of the little toe for 6 to 8 minutes.
(2) The area at the root of the big toe nail for 2 minutes.

Retroversion of the Uterus
Moxa the tip of the process of the 5th lumbar vertebra for 5 minutes. If possible, also needle VC 3.

Frigidity/Impotence
Treatment is bilateral at a point on the abdomen, $\frac{1}{2}$ *tsun* from the medial line, and midway between VC 7 and VC 8. Moxa for 4 to 6 minutes. If possible, also needle VC 7.

Sprained Ankle
Two bilateral points may be treated:

(1) The tip of the internal malleolus.
(2) The centre of the posterior edge of the heel, at the edge of the plantar skin.

Moxa for a total treatment time of 8 to 12 minutes. If possible also prick and bleed the point of the external malleolus.

Lumbar Pains
When these pains are caused by prolonged standing, treat with moxa at a point lateral to BL 47, and $4\frac{1}{2}$ *tsun* from the medial line. Treatment time is 10 to 12 minutes.

Sciatica
Moxa for 8 to 10 minutes at the tip of the process of the 5th lumbar vertebra. If possible also needle a special point .4 *tsun* above BL 60.

Shoulder Articulation Difficulty
Treat with moxa at *Chientungtien*, which is at the middle of the lateral border of the scapula, for 10 to 20 minutes. If there is difficulty in raising the arm, apply moxibustion at a point at the end of the acromion between CO 15 and CO 16 for 5 to 10 minutes.

Spinal Deformation
Use moxa bilaterally at points .8 *tsun* at each side of GV 6 for 15 to 20 minutes.

Knee Weakness
Moxa the apex of the patella, and ST 35, for 3 minutes.

Eye Conditions
Moxa a point at the edge of each thumb, level with LU 10 for 4 to 6 minutes. This point is at the junction of the *Yin* and *Yang* skins.

Toothache
Toothache may be treated with moxa at the feet:

(1) The tip of the internal malleolus.
(2) Along the webs of the toes from LI 2 to GB 43.

Total treatment time for both feet is 10 to 15 minutes.

An additional point for pain in the upper jaw is at the point of the ulnar styloid at the wrist, just proximal to SI 5. For pain in the lower jaw, use a point midway between PC 5 and PC 6. There is no time limit to the treatment of the latter points, which may be used unilaterally when the toothache is at one side of the mouth. Treat the left wrist for pain on the right side, and vice versa.

Boils
Treat with moxa at two unilateral points, left side for men, right side for women.

(1) A special point on the heart meridian, $\frac{1}{4}$ *tsun* above the wrist flexure.
(2) CO 4.

Frequent 5 minute treatments are recommended.

Paralysis, especially Hemiplegia
Treatment commits both acupuncturist and patient to prolonged and painstaking treatment. Treat with moxa two bilateral points:

(1) The posterior aspect of the external malleolus, between the tip of the malleolus and BL 60.
(2) The point of the styloid of the ulna, about $\frac{1}{2}$ *tsun* above SI 5.

No limit can be suggested as to the frequency and duration of the treatment.

8

Electronic Acupuncture

There are now many varieties of electronic acupuncture instruments available. They have one or more of the following functions:

Point Location
Usually the patient holds á metal electrode in one hand, while the acupuncturist moves a probe over the surface of the skin to locate the required point. This forms an electrical circuit in which the point location instrument measures the variations in the current. The electrical resistance of the acupuncture points is less than the resistance of the surrounding area. So the current is increased at these points. The increased current is usually indicated by a change in the sound made by the instrument.

Diagnosis
This is usually an extension of the point location function. The patient holds the hand electrode. The instrument is set to give a meter reading instead of producing a sound. The acupuncturist notes the reading of the meter at a selected point on each meridian, usually at the wrist and ankle. Comparison of the readings with a standard scale indicates which meridians are in excess, and which are deficient, in energy.

Treatment
Instruments for therapy usually have several outlet points. A pair of wire leads may be plugged into each socket. Each pair of wires terminates in two small clips which are attached to the needles after they have been inserted into the skin. The current to each outlet can be regulated separately. If needles are not to be used, small electrodes may be taped to the skin, over the acupuncture point.

These three functions are sometimes incorporated into one instrument. More often the instrument is designed for point location and treatment. This is not an entirely satisfactory

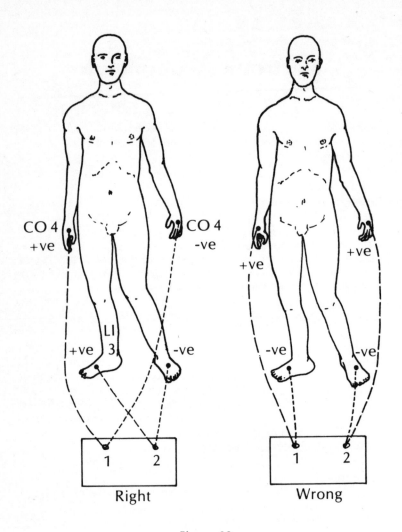

Figure 32

combination because the point locator is ideally as compact as possible, and the therapy instrument should be big enough to provide large, easily-adjusted control knobs. For this reason a separate pen-sized locator is well worth the slight extra cost.

An ideal therapy instrument would have low-geared large knobs to control the strength of the current. Preferably these would be capable of being placed under the control of the patient. Many patients are scared of an electric current which is gradually being increased, however much the acupuncturist assures them that he will stop as soon as the patient tells him it is uncomfortable. The degree of stimulation which the patient finds bearable, and that which is painful and frightening, is often the merest fraction of a degree on a tiny knob on a badly designed instrument. Some otherwise admirable instruments are almost useless because of badly-designed controls. Test any instrument on yourself before you buy it.

Advantages of Electronic Acupuncture
(1) Electronic stimulation shortens the time of treatment. 5 to 10 minutes stimulated, is often the equivalent of 20 to 30 minutes unstimulated.
(2) It often reduces the number of treatments necessary.
(3) It gives a clearly-defined sedation (draining) or tonification (stimulation) effect.

Needleless Electronic Acupuncture
Electronic stimulation of the electrodes taped to the skin may be substituted for needle acupuncture in most cases (see Chapter Six). The most interesting development in needleless acupuncture is the use of laser beams. The potential for this form of acupuncture appears to be enormous, but it is beyond the scope of this book at this time.

The Connection of Electrodes
The following rules apply to both needle and skin electrodes:

Rule One: Try to keep the polarity of the electrodes to the same side of the body, i.e., all positive (usually red) on one side of the body, and all negative (usually black) on the other side. There is an important exception to this rule:

Rule Two: Disregard Rule One only when electrodes are used on the trunk above the level of *Mingmen* (GV 4). A current should not be passed directly through the body above this level, so all electrodes above this line should be of the same polarity (see Figure 33).

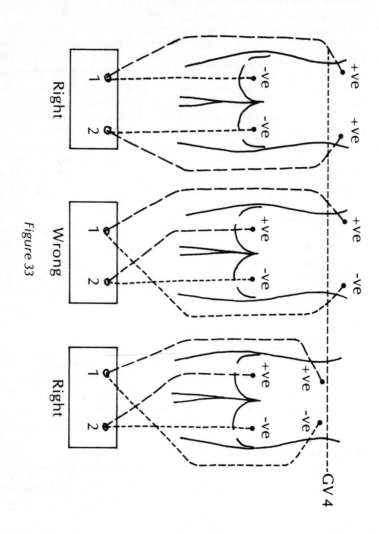

Figure 33

Note that in *Example A*, the points GB 25 are above the level of GV 4. Both electrodes above this level must be of the same polarity, in this case positive.

Example B, shows the electrodes connected under rule one, which is wrong in this case.

Example C, shows the electrodes again connected under rule one. As all electrodes are below the level of GV 4, this is now correct.

Rule Three: Avoid having two electrodes from the same outlet in the same ear. The best arrangement is to connect one electrode to the ear, and the other to body, arm or leg point. An acceptable alternative is to have the positive electrode to one ear, and the negative to the other ear (see Figure 34).

Rule Four: Never use electrical stimulation to needles in the heart meridian. A low current of only 20 micro-volts can be fatal if passed through the heart.

Note that *Example A* shows the correct way of connecting one ear acupuncture point. The negative electrode is connected to any suitable body point, or to a hand-held electrode.

Example B shows two points in the same ear connected to two outputs. The negative leads go to body points. It would be *incorrect* to take a positive and negative lead from one output to the two ear points.

Example C. It is acceptable to connect the positive lead to a point in the right ear, and the negative lead to different acupuncture point in the left ear.

Wave Forms

There are two forms of electric current, direct and alternating. Both may be used for therapy, but the direct current, which is also known as d.c. or galvanic, is rarely used in connection with acupuncture. The effect of direct current is worth noting however, because the form of alternating current produced by many acupuncture instruments has a noticable positive bias. Such a current acts, to some extent, as if it were a direct current, but without the dangers which exist with d.c.

Direct Current

A direct, or galvanic current flows one way, from negative to positive. One electrode is always positive, and the other is negative.

The current only has an effect, from the point of view of therapy, when it is being switched on, or switched off. i.e.,

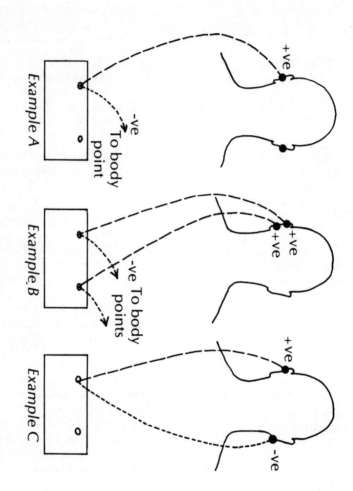

Figure 34

when it is increasing or decreasing in strength. The effect on each electrode is different:

Positive electrode: Sedating, relieves pain. It is acid, and produces a burning sensation.
Negative electrode: Tonifying, improves circulation. It is alkaline, and produces a feeling of numbness or stinging.

Galvanic current, if used at all, may be used for a second or two, only. Otherwise serious internal chemical burns, which may last for years, can be caused. The wave patterns are sawtooth or ripple (see Figure 35a).

Alternating Current
Alternating, or faradic, current changes direction rapidly. Both electrodes are positive and negative in turn. The current flows in each direction for only a fraction of a second, and can therefore be relatively strong without causing damage or distress.

If more current flows on the positve cycle than on the negative cycle, there is an additional galvanic effect. This produces slight sedation at the positive-biased electrode, and slight tonification at the negative-biased electrode. This polarity is the result of a greater pulse-width on the positive cycle (see Figure 35b).

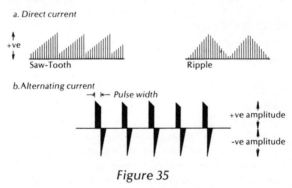

Figure 35

The frequency of the alternating current is the rate at which it changes direction. This is expressed in Hz or Hertz, which is the number of cycles per second. Figure 35b represents 4 cycles. If these took place in one second, the frequency of the current would be 4 Hz.

On any acupuncture instrument, the frequency of the current can be adjusted. In many cases the instrument can be adjusted to send out pulses at a set frequency, alternating with short periods when no current is being sent out. This is called an intermittent current. The patterns of current in common use are:

Dispersed Regular
Frequency about 2 Hz. It has the effect of tonification. It increases the threshold of pain, which tends to remain at the higher level. For chronic pain, numbness, strokes, paralysis, itching skin. Pulse is usually light, and the tongue is white.
   Tune to threshold of perception only.
   Treat 15 to 20 minutes.

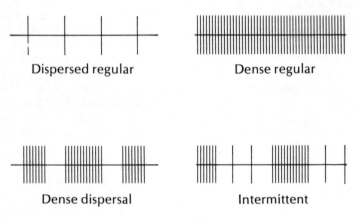

Dispersed regular   Dense regular

Dense dispersal   Intermittent

Figure 36

Dense Regular
Frequency of 50 to 200 Hz. It has the effect of sedation. Mainly for the relief of pain. It increases the pain threshold, but this effect may not be long-lasting. The patient quickly becomes tolerant to the dense regular frequency, and the setting may need to be turned-up every one or two minutes.
   Tune to the threshold of pain.
   Treat 15 to 30 minutes.

Intermittent
Gives good relief from pain, but patients often find it uncomfortable. A more satisfactory pattern combines dispersed-regular with dense-regular intermittantly. This is known as dense-dispersal.

Dense-dispersal
This is the best general-purpose frequency pattern. Short periods of dispersed-regular are followed by short periods of dense-regular. Most patients find it fairly comfortable, and tolerance does not build up too quickly.
   Tune to threshold of pain.
   Treat 15 to 30 minutes.

Duration and Intensity of Treatments
The upper and front parts of the body, and the elbow and knee areas are more conductive than the lower and back parts of the body.
   The less-conductive areas need longer and more intensive therapy than the more-conductive areas (see Figure 37).

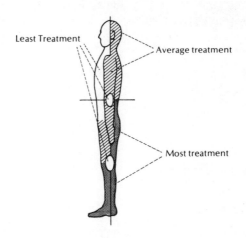

Figure 37

Specific Treatments for Electronic Needle Acupuncture

To Give Up Smoking
Treat Lung and Shenmen points in the ear, three times per week. Use regular-dense current at 125 Hz for 20 minutes. When treating the lung point, avoid the heart point itself, as use of this may increase blood pressure.

To Control Appetite
Treat hunger, Shenmen, stomach and mouth points in the ear. All points may be used, or hunger plus the most sensitive of the other three.

Treat twice weekly with 3-5 minutes dense, plus 5 to 10 minutes dense-dispersal. Leave press needle in hunger. Use alternate ears each visit.

Hunger is an area rather than a point. Use a point detector to locate the most sensitive spot on the centre of the tragus.

If patient suffers from fluid retention, leave a second press needle in the most sensitive spot in the area immediately below the hunger point.

Alcoholism

Treat liver point in the ear, with dense-regular current at 125 Hz, three times weekly, for 30 minutes.

Asthma

Treat lung and asthma 2 points in the ear, bilaterally with dense-dispersal, twice weekly for 20 to 30 minutes.

Further Reading

The Acupuncture Treatment of Pain
  Leon Chaitow
The Complete Book of Acupuncture
  Dr S.T. Chang
The Complete Guide to Acupuncture
  Masaru Toguchi
Essentials of Acupuncture
  Dr Henry Voisin
Japanese Acupuncture
  Mme Dr M. Hashimoto
The Little Red Book of Acupuncture
  Dr Jean-Paul Leger

Index